Back to Work for the Breastfeeding Mother

Excerpt from Working and Breastfeeding Made Simple

Nancy Mohrbacher, IBCLC, FILCA

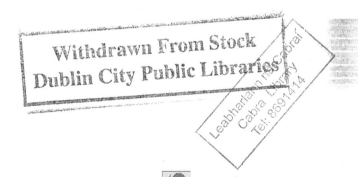
Praeclarus Press, LLC
©2016 Nancy Mohrbacher. All rights reserved.

www.PraeclarusPress.com

Praeclarus Press, LLC
2504 Sweetgum Lane
Amarillo, Texas 79124 USA
806-367-9950
www.PraeclarusPress.com

DISCLAIMER
The information contained in this publication is advisory only and is not intended to replace sound clinical judgment or in-dividualized patient care. The author disclaims all warranties, whether expressed or implied, including any warranty as the quality, accuracy, safety, or suitability of this information for any particular purpose.

ISBN: 978-1-939807-47-2
©2014 Nancy Mohrbacher. All rights reserved.

Cover Design: Ken Tackett
Acquisition & Development: Kathleen Kendall-Tackett
Copy Editing: Diana Cassar-Uhl, Chris Tackett
Layout & Design: Nelly Murariu
Operations: Scott Sherwood

Table of Contents

1

Intro

If you're reading this, chances are you are planning (or have already begun) to work and breastfeed. Why do you need this book? First, you'll find tips and insights that can simplify your life and make the process less confusing. Second, despite the glut of available information, without some inside knowledge, you're unlikely to meet your breastfeeding goals. I chose this book's content to help you avoid the experience of most women. A 2012 study found that two thirds of American mothers who wanted to exclusively breastfeed for three months didn't (Perrine, Scanlon, Li, Odom, & Grummer-Strawn, 2012).

Employed mothers—especially those working full time—are even less likely to reach their breastfeeding targets than other mothers (Ogbuanu, Glover, Probst, Hussey, & Liu, 2011). In every developed country around the world, breastfeeding rates drop quickly after birth. Even in areas where new mothers receive many months of paid maternity leave, such as the U.K., breastfeeding rates plummet during the early weeks. But before I say more about the challenges and how this book can help you avoid and overcome them, I'd like to share with you the latest on why breastfeeding matters so much to you and your baby.

Why Breastfeeding Matters

Most mothers know that babies who are not breastfed are at greater risk for many health problems. But only recently have we begun to understand the risk to mothers when breastfeeding is cut short. Breastfeeding is not just important to your baby. It's also important to you.

Breastfeeding and You

Breastfeeding is a key women's health issue. A growing body of research has linked a lack of breastfeeding and early weaning to the number one killer of women, heart disease, as well as breast and ovarian cancers, metabolic syndrome, type 2 diabetes, and many other serious health problems. Breastfeeding even affects your response to stress (helping you cope with it better), your resistance to illness (boosting it), and how well and how long you sleep (longer and deeper).

For years, people assumed that breastfeeding was draining to mothers. While fatigue is a normal part of life for all new parents, it turns out this assumption was dead wrong. Your body adapts to lactation by reducing the energy required to make milk, which also improves your other body functions. Scientists think that milk-making actually "primes" or "resets" your metabolism after birth to boost your metabolic efficiency (Stuebe & Rich-Edwards, 2009). Lactation improves digestion and increases absorption of nutrients (Hammond, 1997). It increases your sensitivity to the hormone insulin in the short and long term. For every year you breastfeed, over the next 15 years, your risk of developing type 2 diabetes decreases by about 15% (Stuebe, Rich-Edwards, Willett, Manson, & Michels, 2005).

Breastfeeding and Your Baby

Thousands of studies have reported on the health drawbacks when babies are not breastfed. The American Academy of Pediatrics 2012 Policy Statement recommends exclusive breastfeeding for the first six months and a minimum of one year of total breastfeeding (AAP, 2012). Babies who are *not breastfed* are at increased risk of these health problems.

- 72% increased risk of lower respiratory infections
- 63% increased risk of upper respiratory infections

- 50% increased risk of ear infections

- 40% increased risk of asthma

- 42% increased risk of allergic rashes

- 64% increased risk of digestive tract infections

- 30% increased risk of type 1 diabetes

- 36% increased risk of Sudden Infant Death Syndrome

But a healthier first year is not the end of the story. One compelling reason that one year of breastfeeding is recommended is that these health differences are not restricted to infancy. Babies who do not breastfeed or who wean early are more likely to develop the following conditions as they mature: obesity, diabetes, inflammatory bowel diseases, celiac disease, and childhood leukemia and lymphoma. For an overview of why breastfeeding matters from a health standpoint to both you and your baby, see the 2010 article "The Risks and Benefits of Infant Feeding Practices for Women and Their Children" (Stuebe & Schwarz, 2010): _http://www.ncbi.nlm.nih.gov/pmc/articles/PMC2812877/ pdf/RIOG002004_0222.pdf_.

You may find this information disturbing or motivating, but in either case, you need it. In order to make a truly informed decisions, parents need to know how breastfeeding impacts lifelong health. When it comes to breastfeeding, knowledge is definitely power. Knowing what's at stake may help you get through the rough spots that many breastfeeding mothers experience.

For many women, though, the importance of breastfeeding to health isn't even on their radar. Breastfeeding's main appeal is that it increases the connection between mother and baby. When you and your baby are regularly apart, your emotional connection with your baby looms large, as Marge describes.

> I loved that this was something only I could do for my baby. I was worried he would think his nanny was his mom, but everyone reassured me children always know who the mom is—from the intensity of the relationship and connection. Still, the breast-feeding and providing all his milk made me feel connected, a 24/7 mom.
>
> —*Marge G., Ohio, USA*

How can you make breastfeeding—and the close connection that it fosters—a reality? That's what this book is about.

Let Me Be Your Guide

My love for breastfeeding began when I breastfed my own three sons, who are now grown. I started working with mothers as a volunteer in 1982. After I became board-certified, for 10 years, I ran a large private lactation practice in the Chicago area, where I worked one-on-one with thousands of families. I also worked for eight years as a lactation consultant for a major breast pump company, educating health care providers and answering mothers' questions about milk supply and how to make the most of a breast pump. I wrote breastfeeding books used worldwide by parents and professionals, which has kept me current in the lactation research. When I began writing this book, I worked in a corporate lactation program, where I talked daily to women who were pregnant, on maternity leave, and who had returned to work. As you can probably tell, I have a passion for helping breastfeeding mothers. I'd love to share what I've learned with you.

In this book, I've included the key ingredients that make breastfeeding work. It's not complicated. In fact, much of it is very simple. But without this information, working and breastfeeding may be more difficult or more worrisome than it needs to be. These pages include the latest on many of the burning issues you may face: milk production, maternity leave, pumping, flexible job options, childcare, milk storage and handling, work-life balance, and much, much more.

But before we get into these specifics, let me circle back to the sobering figures I mentioned in the beginning on how many women wean earlier than intended. I'd like to explain some of the dynamics that affect these numbers.

The Challenges in Brief

Why is breastfeeding so challenging for so many mothers? One reason is that many mothers and babies don't get the help they need from the institutions that touch their lives. For example, the U.S. Centers for Disease Control and Prevention report that after birth, one in every four U.S. newborns is supplemented in the hospital with infant formula (Centers for Disease Control and Prevention, 2012). Giving newborns formula unnecessarily is a common first step to milk-production problems. Science tells us that worry about milk production is the number one reason women wean before they'd planned. Because many health professionals receive no breastfeeding training, they often give mothers conflicting advice while they are still in the hospital. And some of this advice undermines mothers' best efforts to breastfeed.

After mother and baby arrive home, if breastfeeding problems develop, skilled help is not always affordable or easy to find. When maternity leave ends, many women find their workplaces lack the support they need to continue breastfeeding.

At this writing, the U.S. health care law, the Affordable Care Act, is now in place. According to this law, the costs of breastfeeding supplies and services for new mothers should be covered by health insurance.

How this law's provisions will translate into reality is still unclear. As always, the devil is in the details.

Weaning earlier than intended, however, is not always the result of health care or worksite challenges. It has a much more personal side. Another major reason so many women stop nursing before they had planned is that they are confused about what's normal and how breastfeeding works (DaMota, Banuelos, Goldbronn, Vera-Beccera, & Heinig, 2012). My hope is that this book will provide an antidote to this confusion so that you can experience the empowerment that comes from reaching your breastfeeding goals.

Maternity Leave

The length of your maternity leave is a big piece of this puzzle. Paid maternity leave is available in almost every country, but the details vary from place to place. In Sweden, for example, one year of paid maternity leave is standard, and fathers also have six months of paid leave. In Canada, depending on how long a mother has been at her job and how many hours per week she works, she may be eligible for 15 weeks of paid leave at full salary with an option to take up to 52 weeks at partial salary and her job guaranteed. Yet not all Canadian mothers take advantage of this.

In the U.K., mothers receive 90% of their weekly salary for the first six weeks after birth and the option of up to 52 weeks maternity leave. After the first six weeks, they can stay home at a flat rate for the next 33 weeks, and the last 13 weeks are unpaid. In Australia, 12 months unpaid leave is guaranteed, and the Australian government pays employers (who pass this on to mothers) up to 18 weeks of pay at the national minimum wage, in addition to whatever job benefits mothers receive. But even where paid maternity leave is available, some women do not take advantage of it.

In the United States, under the Family and Medical Leave Act, 12 weeks of unpaid leave is the law of the land, but that's only for those working full time in companies with more than 50 employees. For many American women, any maternity leave—paid or unpaid—is just a dream. But because maternity leave in the U.S. is tied to job benefits, some have more leeway than others. Women employed at the upper levels of large corporations may receive six months or more of paid leave, while women in low-income jobs may have no leave at all and be forced by money pressures to return to work within weeks—or even days—after giving birth.

How This Book Can Help

No matter where you live or what kind of work you do, knowing how the length of your maternity leave affects your back-to-work planning may give you a useful perspective. Even if you have no say in your maternity leave, these insights will give you a better idea of what to expect. Hopefully, having this big picture will help you put the sometimes-confusing details into place.

My fondest hope is that this book will help you achieve your personal breastfeeding goals. Especially during the early weeks, breastfeeding can sometimes feel like a marathon. But like a marathon, crossing the finish line can be a real peak experience. And like the effort that goes into preparing for a race, the more you put into your breastfeeding relationship, the more you can relish the elation that comes with such an outstanding achievement. Between now and then, I'll be cheering you on.

Nancy Mohrbacher
Arlington Heights, IL USA

2

Transition to Work

Do you wonder when you should start preparing in earnest for your return to work? This chapter offers some guidance on when to begin freezing milk, how much milk to store, and how to calculate the milk your baby will need during your work day. Since your top priority while on leave is to enjoy this time with your baby, you also need to know how to keep pumping to a minimum without shortchanging your back-to-work planning. This chapter also explores whether or not you will be pumping at work, and your options either way. It also provides practical tips on scheduling, pumping shortcuts, and even your work wardrobe.

Freezing Milk for Work

How can you balance your time with your baby with your need to prepare for work? Let's start with some pumping strategies.

Pumping During Maternity Leave

While on maternity leave, many mothers spend too much time pumping. How much is too much? Perhaps a better understanding of the basics will explain.

Time to Practice

If you'll be pumping at work, try to allow at least three to four weeks of practice with your pump before your first day back. It takes time to condition your body to release your milk to the pump like it does to your baby. And this conditioning will be much easier to do while you're at home, where you can nurse the baby if the pump does not drain you well.

When to Start Storing Milk

If you feel pressure to start pumping and storing right after birth, take a few deep breaths. There are drawbacks to pumping too early. One is the low return on investment. During the first month—when your milk production is ramping up—you will pump much less milk than you will later. If you're exclusively breastfeeding, pump average amounts of milk, and are pumping between feedings, at one week, your milk yield from both breasts is likely to be around 0.75 oz. (22.5 mL). By four weeks or so, an average pump session between feedings yields more like 1.5 to 2 oz. (45-60 mL), which gives you much more milk in the same amount of time. Unless you're starting back to work before six weeks, you may want to wait. You will get far more milk for your freezer stash if you wait until your baby is at least three to four weeks old to start pumping and storing.

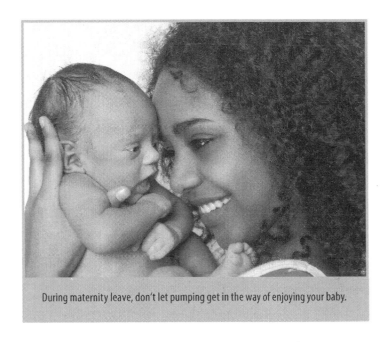

During maternity leave, don't let pumping get in the way of enjoying your baby.

What if you're returning to work much later? If you'll be starting work before your baby is about 9 months old and you want to store milk for your work days, allow about one month to build a healthy freezer reserve. For more details, see the next section.

Variables to Consider

Your pumping plan at home will depend in part on the length of your maternity leave, whether or not you plan to exclusively breastfeed, your work schedule, and whether or not you'll be pumping at work (a later section covers this last option).

Not exclusively breastfeeding. If you don't plan to exclusively breastfeed after returning to work, you can pump or not pump at home as you choose. Your pumping decisions will depend on your baby's age and how much of your milk you want to have on hand after you're back at work (see next section). If your baby will be older than 12 months when you start work, this is not a burning issue, as most employed mothers have stopped pumping by then anyway. While you're at work, babies older than 1 year can drink other milks and liquids, although your baby would certainly benefit from continuing to receive your milk if you choose.

What if your baby is younger than 1 year and you plan to provide your milk exclusively? See where you fit among the following categories.

Full-time job, baby younger than 6 months, exclusively breastfeeding. If you plan to provide your milk only for your younger baby, keep in mind that, very likely, you will pump enough milk at work each day to provide what your baby needs for the following day. When you're at work and missing feedings, expect to pump twice the milk you pump at home between feedings.

How much frozen milk should you have stored when you go back to work? Some of this depends on your comfort level. Will you feel anxious if you start work with less than a whole freezer full of milk? Or would you be happy to start work with just enough milk to cover the first day?

A good middle ground is to plan to have enough frozen milk for your first day back and some extra to cover the unexpected. If you and your baby are average, this would be about 12 oz. (360 mL) for the first day plus another 10 feedings of 3 to 4 oz. (90 to 120 mL) each. But you get to decide what feels right to you. If you're average and you pump once in the morning every day during the month before you return to work, that's about how much milk you'll accumulate.

If you'll be returning to work before your baby is 6 weeks old, you may need to begin pumping earlier and more often. In this case, since you'll be away from your baby during the time she would be breastfeeding intensively to stimulate a full milk supply, more intensive pumping can help you get there sooner. Although your pump yields may be low, pumping after at least three to four feedings each day and evening should boost milk production. (You need your sleep at night to recover from childbirth.) And you can combine these small batches of milk and freeze them for later. Make sure you're draining your breasts well with the baby or the pump at least 8 to 12 times per day until you reach full milk production, which is about 30 oz. (900 mL) per day.

Full-time job, baby older than 6 months, providing your milk only. As babies eat more solid foods, they need less milk. A baby in the 6-to-8-month age range will still need either mother's milk or formula for much of her intake during the work day. Some babies are slow to take solids. In this case, use as a starting point the volumes mentioned in the previous situation: 12 oz. (360 mL) for the first day of work plus another 10 or 15 feedings of 3 to 4 oz. (90 to 120 mL) each. Again, adjust according to your own comfort level.

If your baby is 9 to 12 months old, again with the addition of more solid foods, she will need less milk.

> What's a good freezer stash goal? If you'll be working full-time, aim for 12 oz. (360 mL) for the first day of work plus as a reserve for the unexpected, another 10 or so feedings of 3 to 4 oz. (90 to 120 mL) each.

It's also normal for your milk production to decrease as your baby takes more other foods. So don't be surprised if your pumping volumes are lower than before. Because babies' intake of solid food varies so much, it is difficult to predict exactly how much milk your baby will need during this stage.

Part-time job, exclusively breastfeeding. When you work part time, there are many moving parts involved. Your choices will depend on the specifics. Working 10 hours per week is obviously much different than working 30 hours per week. The length of your work day is also important. Will you be working a few long days or many short days? See the final chapter for sample work schedules and plans. Also look at the previous section if you're working full time. Use that as a benchmark and adjust downward accordingly.

When and How Often to Pump at Home

If you're returning to work after 6 weeks, the good news is that you don't need to pump often to build a healthy freezer stash.

"..it only takes 1 daily pumping for a month to build a healthy reserve of milk."

How often to pump. If your baby is older than 6 weeks and your goal is to store maybe 12 oz. (360 mL) for the first day back and 10 more feedings in your freezer, it only takes 1 daily pumping for a month to build a healthy reserve of milk. If you're pumping between feedings and you get the expected half a feeding per pump session, pumping once a day for 30 days equals 15 feedings. Again, if you'll be pumping at work, you will likely be able to pump enough milk there each day for the next day's feedings. Your reserve is there to cover the unexpected.

When to pump. While you're on leave, to avoid upsetting your baby or shortchanging her need for milk, try to allow at least an hour between pumping and breastfeeding. On average, babies only take about two-thirds of the milk that's in the breast, so there is usually milk left to express after a feeding (Kent, 2007). If you wait a little while before pumping, you'll get even more milk. Try these tips:

- Pump in the morning, as most women get more milk then than later in the day.

- Pump 30 to 60 minutes after a breastfeeding.

Another option is to pump one breast while your baby breastfeeds from the other breast. This works especially well if your baby usually takes one breast per feeding.

If your baby wants to breastfeed right after you pump, go ahead. Most babies are patient and don't mind feeding longer. Your baby can go back and forth from breast to breast several times if needed. Milk is constantly being produced, so even if you just finished pumping, there will be milk for your baby.

Your Baby's Milk Needs During the Work Day

To calculate your baby's milk needs during the work day, let's first focus on the bigger picture. Typically, milk production reaches its peak at about 5 weeks and stays remarkably stable until about 6 months (Kent et al., 2013). At 6 months, as your baby takes more solid foods, her need for milk decreases.

Your Baby's 24-Hour Milk Intake

On average, 1-to-6-month-old breastfed babies consume about 30 oz. (900 mL) of milk per 24-hour day. However, not every baby is average. Some breastfed babies gain weight well on much less milk; others on much more. One study measured 24-hour milk intake in 71 thriving exclusively breastfed babies and found their daily milk intake ranged from 16 oz. (480 mL) to 42 oz. (1220 mL). That's a huge range! Some took almost triple the milk of others. What this means to you is that you don't need to panic if the 30-oz. (900 mL) average does not seem right for your baby. What's most important is that your baby has a healthy weight gain, which is about 1 oz. (30 g) per day for the first three months and less as baby gets older.

That said, let's use the 30-oz. (900 mL) average as a benchmark for calculating your baby's need for milk during your work day. It will quickly become obvious if these numbers are off, and you can adjust if needed. For example, most breastfed babies take on average 3 to 4 oz. (90 to 120 mL) of milk per feeding, which is a good place to start when choosing your batch size. But some babies take more and others take less. Sarah C., a holistic health practitioner from Illinois, USA, discovered to her surprise when she returned to work full-time at seven weeks, that her baby never took more than 2.5 oz. (75 mL) at a feeding. Until you're sure how much milk your baby wants, you may want to start with smaller volumes and store some 1 and 2 oz. (30 and 60 mL) batches to add as needed.

Calculating Your Baby's Milk Needs

When calculating how much milk your baby needs while you're at work, ask yourself these questions.

How many hours are you apart, including travel time? And how much of the 24-hour day is that? For example, if you're away from your baby for eight hours, that is one third of the 24-hour day. One third of 30 oz. (900 mL) is 10 oz. (300 mL). The points below list several time frames and the average milk volumes you should expect your baby to need.

- 6 hours apart (one quarter of a 24-hour day) one quarter of 30 oz.(900 mL) is 7.5 oz. (250 mL)

- 8 hours apart (one third of a 24-hour day) one third of 30 oz. (900 mL) is 10 oz. (300 mL)

- 12 hours apart (half of a 24-hour day) half of 30 oz. (900 mL) is 15 oz. (450 mL)

Again, keep in mind that your baby will need about the same amount of milk per day at 5 weeks as he will at 6 months. Unlike the baby who is formula-fed, breastfed babies do not need more and more milk as they grow bigger and heavier because as they grow, their rate of growth slows (Kent et al., 2013; Kent et al., 2006).

Does your baby breastfeed during the night? This is important to know, too. The calculations above are based on your baby breastfeeding around the clock. However, if you have an unusual baby who sleeps for stretches longer than 4 to 6 hours, you need to calculate differently. For example, if your baby sleeps eight hours straight at night, this means she needs to consume all 30 oz. (900 mL) of her daily milk intake within the 16 hours she's awake. That's a very different equation! Because eight hours is half of your baby's 16-hour feeding day, this means that for an eight-hour work day, your baby will need half of her daily intake, or 15 oz. (450 mL). If you're apart for 12 hours, this is three-quarters of her waking hours, and she'll need three-quarters of her milk intake, or slightly more than 22 oz. (660 mL). Big difference!

Pumping at Work: Will You or Won't You?

Pumping at home is one thing, but do you wonder if pumping at work makes sense for you? If so, you're not alone. Before deciding whether to pump at work, it's wise to consider the pros and cons. Here are some points to consider.

Work Pumping Advantages

If your baby is younger than 1 year, isn't available to breastfeed during work, and you work long days, there are benefits to pumping at work.

- It keeps you comfortable and prevents the embarrassment of leaking milk.

- It decreases your risk of painful breast problems, such as mastitis.

- It helps maintain your milk production.

- It avoids some or all of the cost and health issues associated with the use of infant formula.

Work Pumping Challenges

Of course, pumping at work is not all sweetness and light. There are also downsides.

- It takes time away from work, which may involve arriving early or staying late to make up for lost work time.

- It reduces time spent socializing during breaks and meals.

- It requires finding a comfortable, private, easily accessible place to pump.

- It may mean dealing with push-back from employers or coworkers.

When considering your options, keep in mind that like breastfeeding, pumping doesn't have to be all or nothing. Even if you can't or don't want to pump the ideal number of times per day, some pumping is always an option.

Pumping Is Temporary

Keep in mind, too, nearly all mothers stop pumping at work by or around their baby's first birthday. How long you decide to pump at work, of course, depends on your unique situation, as well as your baby's age. If your baby is a year or older, pumping might not even be on your radar. If pumping is part of your experience, however, don't forget that the need to pump is temporary. Knowing this may make it feel more manageable to both you and your employer.

If You Won't Be Pumping at Work

Much of this book describes strategies for mothers who pump at work. But if you don't plan to pump, you need strategies, too. You may wonder, for example, if you must wean completely to avoid painful breast fullness and leaking milk at work. The answer is no. You have a number of other options, as well. This section gives you tips for maximizing breastfeeding during your maternity leave while safeguarding your comfort and sanity after you return to work. It even includes options other than weaning.

Weighing Feeding Options

You may be surprised to know that even if you're working full-time and won't be pumping at work, you still have several options. Some are dependent, though, on where you fall on the breast-storage-capacity spectrum.

The Impact of Breast Storage Capacity

Breast storage capacity is a physical attribute that varies greatly among mothers. Simply put, storage capacity is determined by the amount of milk your breasts contain during their fullest time of the day. It is based not on breast size, but on how much room there is in your milk-making glands. This individual difference has a major implications for employed mothers.

What is its effect? If your capacity is very large, you may be able to go through an entire eight-hour work day without breastfeeding or pumping, yet not suffer any negative consequences. This is rare, but I worked with a mother who did this successfully for four months. She breastfed when she and her baby were together, and was able to pump enough milk before and after work to provide exclusive mother's milk feeds for her baby while she was gone.

Although this worked for her, if your storage capacity is medium or small, your experience would likely be very different. For most mothers, staying very full of milk for eight hours could bring on the breast pain and swelling known as mastitis. Over time, it would also reduce milk supply. (Full breasts make milk slower.) This same approach could produce vastly different outcomes in different women.

How do you know where you fall on the breast-storage-capacity spectrum? You can't know exactly, but there are some clues that can help guide you as you weigh your choices.

What's Your Capacity?

Three aspects of your experience provide clues to your place on this spectrum.

Maximum milk pumped. One obvious indicator is your pumping history, specifically the most milk you've ever expressed in one sitting. Table 1 reflects the experiences of many breastfeeding mothers I have known. It is not based on research, but rather on observation. I hope this can be used as a starting point for others to look at this more scientifically.

Table 1. Breast Storage Capacity Clues

	Largest Capacity	Large Capacity	Medium Capacity	Small Capacity	Smallest Capacity
Max milk pumped	10-15 oz. (300-450 mL)	5-9 oz. (150-270 mL)	3-5 oz. (90-150 mL)	2-3 oz. (60-90 mL)	1-2 oz. (30-60 mL)
# feeds/ day	5-6	6-7	7-8	8-9	≥9
Longest stretch	10-12 hr	8-10 hr	8 hr	6-7 hr	4-5 hr

Have you ever heard of a mother pumping 10 to 15 oz. (300 to 450 mL) in the morning before her baby awakens? This is one sign of a very large breast storage capacity. Some mothers, on the other hand, pump no more than 3 or 4 oz. (90 to120 mL), even when they feel really full. This is the sign of a medium or small storage capacity.

Feeding pattern. If your maternity leave is at least six weeks long and you're exclusively breastfeeding, you may get a sense of your storage capacity from your baby's feeding pattern. After the first month, if your baby is gaining weight well on fewer than eight feedings per day, this may indicate a large capacity. Another aspect of your baby's feeding pattern that provides a clue is whether your baby usually takes one or both breasts per feeding. Typically, babies take both breasts at least some of the time. But mothers with a large storage capacity often report that their babies are almost always satisfied with just one breast.

Longest stretch between feedings. The breastfed babies who sleep for long stretches at night often have mothers with a large breast storage capacity. That's because with so much room in their milk-making glands, their milk production doesn't slow when their babies sleep for longer than six or seven hours at a time. As a side note, it is common for breastfed babies to wake much more often than every four to five hours when they are hungry. This indicator alone does not tell the whole story.

Your Choices

So where does this leave you in terms of options? Here are some things to consider.

Very large storage capacity. If all the indicators tell you that you probably have a large breast storage capacity, this gives you more options than other mothers. If your capacity is very large, you might be able to work full-time and do what the mother whom

I mentioned earlier did. She got up in the morning and pumped milk at home before her baby awakened, which provided most of the milk needed for her work day. Then she breastfed her baby, went to work, and after she returned to her baby at the end of her eight-hour work day, she breastfed again. A pump session shortly after provided the rest of what her baby needed for the next day.

Any size breast storage capacity. The option above will not work for most mothers working full time or long days, so what are some other choices?

- Pump like crazy during your maternity leave and amass a giant freezer stash of milk so that your baby receives your milk for as long as possible after your start back to work.

- Do a partial weaning (see next section) to reduce your milk production enough so you're comfortable during your work day without pumping but can still breastfeed at home. While at work, your baby would receive pumped milk, formula, or both.

- Gradually wean from the breast a couple of weeks before you start back to work, substituting stored milk or formula for feedings.

The choice is completely up to you. When considering your options, keep in mind that breastfeeding doesn't have to be all or nothing. From a health stand-point, there is value to both you and your baby in any amount of nursing.

Staying Comfortable at Work

As mentioned, breast storage capacity can have a huge impact on your comfort at work. The larger your storage capacity, the longer it takes for your breasts to feel full and for your milk production to slow. However, even if your storage capacity is medium or small and your work days long, you still may be able to both breastfeed and stay comfortable.

The Length of Your Work Day

Your comfort and risk of leaking milk are dependent on two main factors, your breast storage capacity and the length of your work day. If your work day is shorter than your longest stretch between feedings at home, you should be able to go back to work without making any changes in your milk supply. Let's say you'll be away from your baby for six hours during your work day, and your baby currently sleeps for six hours at night. If you are comfortable for that six-hour stretch of time, you're good to go. Alternatively, if your time away from your baby is eight hours, and you feel full-to-bursting in the rare cases when you've gone for that long, it's best to make some changes before you return to work.

Would a Partial Weaning Help?

If your work day is longer than your baby's longest stretch between feedings at home and you won't be pumping or breastfeeding at work, consider a partial weaning. It allows you to reduce your milk production enough to avoid full breasts during your work day, yet leaves enough milk so you can breastfeed when you're home. For example, instead of being at full milk production, you might reduce your milk supply by half and breastfeed part time.

How to do a partial weaning. There are different ways to go about this. Here's one:

- Note your usual breastfeeding times. About a week or two before returning to work, pick one feeding during the hours you'll be working. (Avoid the first morning feeding when you will likely feel full already.)

- If you have not given formula, and your baby is younger than 12 months, talk to your baby's health care provider about what to substitute for your milk and feed your baby this at the missed breastfeeding.

- Continue feeding this substitute at about the same time each day.

- Give your body at least two to three days before dropping another breastfeeding. If your breasts become full, express just enough milk to feel comfortable and no more. This will slow your milk production gradually, without pain or risk of infection.

- Repeat until you are comfortable without breast-feeding for the entire length of your work day.

Another way to do a partial weaning is to continue offering the breast first at all feedings while you're with your baby and offer the substitute in-between. When your baby regularly takes as much supplement as you would expect him to take during your work day, you are ready.

Quick Tips for an Easier Transition

While you're in the planning stages, consider these strategies to help ease your adjustment back to work.

Scheduling Your Return

When you notify your employer about your return to work, explore the possibility of moving gradually into your ultimate work schedule. Going slower at first may make this adjustment easier for both you and your baby. Here are some approaches.

Work Fewer Hours Per Week

Whether you'll be working full-time or part-time, consider starting back to work at fewer hours per week for as long as is practical. If your work day is normally 8 hours, see if you can arrange to work four hours per day in the beginning. Then move up to 6 hours per day and eventually increase to your full eight-hour work days. Finances and flexibility will no doubt play a role in how this plays out, but even a short ramp-up may smooth out this process as you adjust.

Schedule a Day Off Mid-week

For example, if you work Monday through Friday, arrange for a while to have Wednesdays off. This gives you a break every two days for rest and catch-up breastfeeding.

Start Near the End of the Week

Rather than starting on a Monday with five full work days ahead of you, consider starting back on a Thursday or Friday. You can either combine this with the previous strategies or as an alternative to them. Even if this is the only scheduling change you can make, it is well worth it.

Postpone Your Return

Alison B. from Indiana, USA described how postponing her return to work made a difference.

Being ready to go back to work and being ready to leave my baby were not the same thing at all. When I planned my maternity leave, I scheduled it for 8 weeks, not really having any idea what that meant. At 6 weeks, I panicked and wrote my boss an email saying that I was postponing my return until 10 weeks, which he thankfully agreed to.

Pump Planning

The following tips may simplify your pumping routine at work and at home.

Your Pump Schedule at Work

No doubt you've already given some thought to your pumping schedule at work. The number of pump sessions per day needed to keep your milk production steady over the long term will depend on your baby's age, your breast storage capacity, the number of hours you and your baby are apart, and whether you plan to provide only your milk for your baby. It will take some time for you to figure out the routine that works best for you. Until then, however, you need a starting point.

Number of pump sessions at work. To decide how many times to pump at work when you first start back, count how many hours you'll be away from your baby, including travel time. Until you see how your body responds to the changes in routine, try not to go longer than about 3 hours without removing the milk from your breasts. Assuming you'll be breastfeeding as the last thing you do before leaving your baby and the first thing you do when you are reunited, use this plan as a starting point:

- 6 hours apart = 1 pump session (unless your baby is already going for 6-hour stretches between feedings at home)

- 9 hours apart = 2 pump sessions

- 12 hours apart = 3 pump sessions

Time needed per pump session. Most mothers working full-time with young babies pump twice per day and spend less than an hour per day total pumping (Slusser, Lange, Dickson, Hawkes, & Cohen, 2004). Allow at least 20 to 30 minutes per pump session, including clean-up.

Where to store your milk. Depending on the room temperature at work and the length of your work day, you may or may not need to cool your pumped milk. The season and your climate will affect whether or not your milk needs to be cooled while you travel from work to home. As long as you follow the milk storage guidelines, any milk you store at room temperature can be refrigerated and/or frozen later.

If you need to cool your milk, you have several options:

- Pump bag cooler compartment with freezer packs

- Separate cooler bag with freezer packs

- Private or shared refrigerator

Simplifying Washing

You can eliminate the need to clean your pump parts at work by buying enough extra pieces so that you have enough clean sets for every pump session. According to the experts, there's no benefit to sterilizing pump parts after every use (Jones & Tully, 2011). Normal hygiene is fine. (Remember, your milk has antibacterial properties.)

To clean your parts, first rinse all the pieces with milk on them in cool water, wash them in warm, soapy water, then rinse well. With the right number of clean sets, you can do all of the washing at home. If you have a dishwasher, it can do this work for you.

You don't have to buy multiple "pump kits," which can be expensive. You just need enough of the specific pump parts that are washed after each pumping session. Normally, that would not include the pump tubing or the piece that connects the tubing to the pump motor. It would include the milk container (most pumps with carry bags come with extra bottles or you can use milk freezer bags), the pump pieces you hold to your breasts, and any other parts that the milk touches. These parts can usually be ordered individually online.

Pump Packing and Unpacking at Home

Work days are full of details to remember, especially during the morning rush. In some families, to streamline their routine, the mother's partner takes on the responsibility of unpacking the pump and milk after work, storing the milk, cleaning the parts, and repacking the pump for the next day. If you have a partner and he or she is available and willing to do this, it can be a significant contribution to the breastfeeding relationship. This commitment allows you to focus on your baby when you're at home, while someone else handles these pumping details for you.

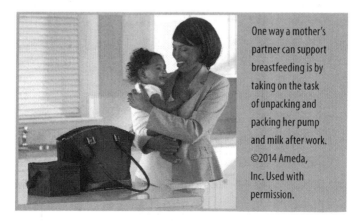

One way a mother's partner can support breastfeeding is by taking on the task of unpacking and packing her pump and milk after work. ©2014 Ameda, Inc. Used with permission.

Work Wardrobe

Before returning to work, think about your wardrobe and how well it fits with your plan to breastfeed or pump. You might also want to consider the following.

- Have breast pads on hand and an extra top available in case of milk leakage. (An alternative is LilyPadz, a silicone product worn inside your bra that applies pressure to your nipples to prevent milk leakage.)

- Wear two-piece outfits, so you can pump or breastfeed without having to fully undress.

- Wear patterned tops rather than solid colors to better camouflage leaks or spilled milk.

- Have a jacket or sweater handy for use as a cover-up if needed.

Now that we've covered many of the practical details of returning to work, it's time to focus on the soft side: your feelings about this major transition and your baby's reaction to your time apart.

3

Your Feelings About Returning to Work

Practical details are important. But feelings are important too. This chapter focuses on the softer side of going back to work: the emotions that go along with it. Mothers' feelings run the gamut, and this chapter covers the entire range. Babies sometimes react to their new back-to-work routine too, most commonly with changes in feeding and sleeping patterns. It can help to know what to expect, and it can most definitely help to know that you're not alone, and where to find the support you need.

What Affects Your Feelings

It's impossible to completely separate your body and your feelings. Both are affected by your return to work.

Physical Recovery

Even at 11 weeks postpartum, many women have not fully physically recovered from delivery. As I described earlier, in one study, women at 11 weeks postpartum reported an average of four childbirth-related symptoms, such as pain and fatigue (McGovern et al., 2007). Mothers who had cesarean sections had more health problems than those who delivered vaginally (McGovern et al., 2006). As Melissa M. from New York, USA described "Six weeks to go through the most life- and body-changing things was a pittance." If you're returning to work within the first three months, expect that it may take awhile for your energy to return to its normal level.

Lauren J. from New York, USA describes her experience: "My son was only 8 weeks old when I had to return to my full-time job as a clinical social worker. It was a tremendous struggle, both physically and emotionally. I felt as though he and I were just starting to get the hang of this breastfeeding thing, and then I had to leave him."

Range of Emotions

Mothers' feelings about returning to work are understandably mixed and vary tremendously from woman to woman.

What Research Tells Us

To understand more fully mothers' feelings about returning to work, researchers surveyed 74 mothers who were back at their full-time jobs after an average of 10 weeks (Nichols & Roux, 2004). Using open-ended questions, the researchers discovered that while the mothers had a variety of feelings, the negatives outweighed the positives. These were the most common challenges women reported. They:

- Found it difficult to leave their babies,

- Felt pressured by conflicting demands on their time and energy,

- Felt overloaded with work-family stresses,

- Faced childcare and financial pressures, and

- Experienced sleep deprivation and mood changes.

On the positive side, these study mothers also:

- Enjoyed motherhood,

- Learned from this experience how to ask for and receive help,

- Successfully realigned their priorities and life-style to better suit their new family dynamics, and

- Derived satisfaction from their work.

Separation Anxiety

The most common challenge the study mothers reported was being separated from their babies. This is not surprising, as a strong emotional attachment to our babies is key to human survival. Rachel F. from Kentucky, USA returned to her full-time job as a public-health counselor at 12 weeks with both of her daughters.

> It doesn't get easier the second time. Both times I didn't want to do it, and both times I cried. Returning to work is one of the hardest things for a mom to experience, in my opinion. When you grow a person inside of you, you instinctively want to remain close to the one who is so dependent on you for everything. Allowing someone else to take care of my girls because I had to work to bring in income for our family was beyond difficult emotionally. I just wanted to be with my babies.

Some mothers find unique ways to cope with this stress. Vivienne M. from Maryland, USA returned to work part time as a software engineer when both of her daughters were 4 months old.

> I was fortunate to be able to telecommute for the first year of their lives, and their caregiver brought them to me when they wanted to feed. (How awesome is that!) When I first returned to work, I re-

member missing my baby physically and feeling guilty that she might be upset and I wasn't there to comfort her. During the first couple of weeks at work, I actually searched around the house, and found a soft toy that was roughly the size of my infant. I tucked it inside my shirt, mimicking the kangaroo position where my baby would sleep, and I felt comforted! I'd tell myself that it was OK to work. The baby was sleeping, and well loved and cared for. Not something that you would want to do in an office, but it just was hard to not have my baby with me, especially during those first couple of weeks.

Some mothers have more mixed feelings about being away from their babies. Becca, A. from Tennessee, USA, returned to work at 12 weeks as a full-time project manager for a publishing house.

I felt very torn at first between enjoying getting back to working life and feeling like part of me was far away. Pumping sessions at work were a break in my day to think about my baby. I would look at pictures and watch videos, and it really brightened my mood and made me miss him less because I was taking breaks to focus on him.

However, once back at work, not all mothers miss their babies. Sofiya P., who worked as a part-time legal secretary for a New York City law firm, was able to work from home for a couple of months, returning to the office three days a week when her baby was 4 months old. She felt relieved to be back in the office.

> Is it strange that I was relieved to go back after 4 months at home with my baby? All I wanted to do was get out of the house, put on clothes that weren't stained or smelled like spit up, and do things that did not involve or revolve around my baby. To this day, I wonder if there is something wrong with me that I don't feel sad dropping my boy off at daycare, where I know he is treated well by kids and caretakers alike. I guess I am lucky that I have a "good" baby. He is social and happy most of the time. When I went back to work, we hired a nanny, and he took to her without a second thought. I found it easier to handle two days at home with him rather than the full work week.

> I wonder how many mothers actually feel the way I do—happy to be doing their job, to be around other adults in a professional setting. You don't see this kind of mother much in the media. Do I wish that I wanted to be home all the time with him? Sometimes. But that is not my reality.

Factors That May Affect Your Feelings

Every mother is different, and there are many factors that may affect how you feel when you start work.

Here are just a few.

- Your job specifics (maternity leave, hours per week, your feelings about your work)

- Your mood and adjustment to motherhood

- Whether your baby is easy, challenging, or in between

Let's look at these factors one by one.

Your job specifics. Many aspects of your job can affect how you feel about returning to it. Does your employer offer much flexibility? Can you leave work at your workplace, or do you have to bring work home? Did you choose to work, or do you have to work? Here are some other factors that may affect your feelings.

A longer maternity leave, usually makes returning to work easier (Ogbuanu, Glover, Probst, Liu, & Hussey, 2011). You have more time to physically recover from childbirth, your baby outgrows the fussy periods that are so common during early infancy, and your months at home make it easier for you and your baby to form a solid bond. Yet a longer maternity leave is no guarantee that you'll feel 100% positive when the time comes to return to work. Michelle P. from Newfoundland, Canada returned to work full-time as a newspaper reporter when her younger daughter was 10 months old.

How did I feel? I felt anxious at first. I wasn't sure how it was going to work out. I dreaded it, honestly. But very quickly I came to feel lucky. At that time, the chaos of two kids at different ages was overwhelming and I was glad to leave that behind for the peace of the office for stretches at a time. I could phone to hear about what was going on and as time went on I really enjoyed the rhythm.

Fionnuala M. from Ireland, a full-time communications manager for a charity, returned to work when her son was 10 months old.

He is my third baby, and I had already worked and breastfed once so I knew I could do it. I knew that my son would survive, but I was worried about how he would manage without the comfort, especially in a new environment. It felt odd to expect him to make such a big adjustment without his daily comfort. Emotionally, I felt a bit conflicted because I wanted to return to work but didn't want to leave my baby, and I was worried about the amount of juggling involved.

Crystal N., a full-time public-health nurse from Manitoba, Canada, returned to work full-time as a public-health nurse when the youngest of her three daughters was 12 months old.

It was very hard to go back after a full year of getting to spend every day with them. I wasn't ready to go back full-time. I felt like I had worked so hard to establish this great breastfeeding team between me and my LO and I couldn't believe it was coming to an end.

The hours per week you work may also influence your feelings. Mothers who work part time breastfeed, on average, as long as mothers who are not employed (Ogbuanu, Glover, Probst, Hussey, & Liu, 2011). Working full time means more hours apart, which often means more breastfeeding challenges. Melissa M. from New York, USA returned to work full time as an education-claims processor for the U.S. Department of Veterans Affairs when her son was 6 weeks and 6 days old.

It was the hardest thing I have ever done. I felt guilty, sad, depressed and without choice. I cried after dropping off, I cried through work, through pumping, and I counted the hours to get back to him. I worked 45 to 50 hours a week when he was tiny. I gave up and went back to refusing overtime as he got older. I didn't want to miss everything to the babysitter/daycare center.

How you feel about your job can also make a difference. If you love your work, you'll probably feel more positively about going back. It's okay to love your baby and your job. Marge G. from Ohio, USA returned to her obstetric practice part time seven weeks after her son Dan was born.

> Dan was nursing well, the pumping was going fine, and I was dying to get back to my "normal life." I loved breastfeeding, and of course I loved my son, but I am not a baby person (funny thing for an OB to say but you know what I mean) and it was so hard being home all day and pacing myself for a baby. I was ready to go back to seeing patients. Fortunately, I had a private administrative office, and my schedule was very flexible, especially since my practice had dwindled while I was out. I blocked out 1.5 hours for lunch/pumping every day around 1 pm, and I could double pump enough for all his feedings during my work day. I was proud of nursing. The breastfeeding and providing all his milk made me feel connected, a 24/7 mother.

Your mood and your adjustment to motherhood. How well you adjust to motherhood and whether you suffer from postpartum depression are likely to affect your feelings too. Karen C. from California, USA worked part time as a technical researcher for an aerospace firm. She describes how her difficult emotional adjustment to motherhood with her first baby affected her feelings about returning to work and how that changed with her second baby.

With my first baby, I couldn't wait to return to work at 4.5 months. My transition to motherhood was difficult emotionally. I felt like a failure as a mother, breastfeeding was a struggle, and she was a higher-needs baby. I looked forward to leaving her with the caregiver that I had worked hard to find, and felt immensely relieved to have three days a week without the stress of being her mother. I noticed that a few hours away from her during the day allowed me the space I needed to let my emotions catch up, and after a few months back at work I began to feel much more bonded than I had before I returned to work. Now she is 4, and I miss her tremendously when we're apart.

My second baby was nothing but joy, an easy birth, natural nurser, an easy-going, happy baby. I dreaded my return to work, also at 4.5 months, and where I had handed my daughter off without a thought, I lingered and lingered at his first drop-off. I missed him terribly.

Depression not only affects a mother's feelings, it can also affect her relationship with her baby and her partner. Joy S. from Kentucky, USA went back to work full-time as a project manager assistant for a general contracting company when her son was 2 months old.

I had a hard time with returning to work. I suffered from postpartum depression, and going back to work did not help. Before he was born, we made the decision that my husband would be a stay-at-home dad. The decision was mainly based on financial reasons. I would have rather been the stay-at-home parent, but I knew logically that this was the best decision for us. My emotions, on the other hand, didn't get that memo! I dealt with jealousy of my husband spending all that time with our son. I felt I was better equipped to be at home and had a hard time letting my husband do things his way. He is a great father and does a great job, but emotionally, it was hard not being at home. It has been an ongoing process of checking my attitude and reminding myself to be thankful that every day I am leaving my son with his father.

An easy or challenging baby. The baby we give birth to is not always the baby we expect. Julianne W. from Connecticut, USA found going back to work hard in part because her daughter Addie was so colicky, which made early motherhood a struggle for her.

For as long as I could remember, I wanted to be a mother. But Addie screamed almost constantly for the first three months of her life. She didn't latch well, didn't sleep well, and generally seemed to hate everything, including me. It was so frustrating and difficult, I cried almost constantly for three months along with her and felt like such a failure. I knew motherhood wouldn't be a walk in a park, but I just wanted to hide in my room or hand Addie over to someone who could obviously do so much better than I was doing. So when returning to work finally came around, I thought it would be pure relief to return to the world of normal volume levels and feeling competent.

But being at work while my husband was at home with a screaming child was terrible for a good while. My husband and I would talk throughout the day and he would tell me how bad the day was going, how cranky Addie was, how she hadn't napped well. This made me feel as if he resented being home (he had worked in a fast-paced office before we moved) and resented me working, even though in his mind, he was simply reporting on the day. The guilt I felt was crippling, causing me to be distracted at work, depressed, and angry with my husband.

For the first month or two after I returned to work, Addie would be screaming when I came home and it was so jarring after a relatively peaceful day that I would take extra time cleaning up my pump parts, stowing my milk, cleaning up the house, and changing my clothes before I could pick her up and say hello. I'm not terribly proud of that, and it made me feel like an even worse mother, especially once my husband realized what was going on and called me out on it. But I also knew that once I was home, I would shoulder 100% of the Addie responsibility as my husband felt like he had already put in his time and it was my turn. And certainly I would want to cuddle up with my child after being away from her all day, right? Yes, but not for the four solid hours before bedtime of screaming, walking around holding her, and feeling once again like a terrible mother who could do no right. And I knew I would sleep with Addie and nurse her several times during the night. It was hard after a draining day at work to be further drained.

Once Addie stopped screaming so much (around 4 or 5 months) and started smiling and interacting, she wanted to be with my husband much more than me, and that really hurt. He's brilliant with her and she adores him for it. It seemed she really only wanted me for milk. I couldn't soothe her when she was crying, or play with her and make her giggle. Then I really felt like a failure, and I was angry with my husband, as if he were turning her against me on purpose. Only recently has she started giving equal "giggle time" and smiles to both mommy and daddy, and I've found ways to soothe her that are my own.

My husband and I are still working through it, and there are still some really bad days. Now that Addie wants to interact, I'm finding new ways to connect with her beyond nursing. It's still hard for me to reconcile my reality with what I thought motherhood would be and feel good about it, but I think we're all finding our groove and figuring out how to be a functional, happier family.

How you feel about your mothering competence (as Julianne's story above illustrates so well) also affects your feelings when you return to work. Your confidence as a mother can be very different with your first baby than with your second. Emily H. from Illinois, USA had her first child when she was 18, just 6 weeks before she started as a full-time college student and began a 20-hour-per-week part-time job. As a first-time mother, she was reluctant to ask for what she needed, which changed with her second baby.

Initially, it was hard. I wasn't quite sure how to make everything work, and I felt guilty and inadequate. I only breastfed my son for about three months, because I didn't pump consistently and my milk supply dropped. Breastfeeding was much easier the second time.

My daughter was born during the fall semester when I was 20, and I took her to my classes. I was pursuing my bachelor's degree in early childhood. Because of my child-development background, I was determined to breastfeed for at least a year. I breastfed on demand for four months, when she started childcare and I returned to work. My milk supply was much more established than it had been with my son, and I was more determined when I returned to my part-time student job. I don't remember feeling guilty as I had with my son. I only felt a determination to ensure I breastfed as long as possible.

I pumped consistently. I was very open with my coworkers, even using a coworker's office to pump during the day. I also was very open with complete strangers. At one point, I had to find another place on campus to pump. I walked into an office filled with women, explained my situation, and they provided me a place to pump when I needed it. I only had to walk into their office and pick up a key.

My first experience with breastfeeding and returning to work was full of disappointment and guilt. I learned from that experience. I was more educated, had more determination, and was successful the second time around.

Breastfeeding Support

Emily's story illustrates how important support can be. One way to reduce the stress of early motherhood and returning to work is to reach out to others. Friends, family, and coworkers may provide support. If you have people in your life who have breastfed as long as you intend to, that's a wonderful thing! But even if you do, there are also other excellent sources of breastfeeding support, both in-person and online. Joy S. from Kentucky, USA, who had suffered with postpartum depression, found breastfeeding-support meetings made a huge difference to her.

> I found and joined a La Leche League group that is a couple of towns over and they have been a tremendous help. There are other working/pumping moms and we compare notes and swap stories. I wish I had found them when I was going through the rough patch, but am very grateful to have them now. I find that I am helping other mothers as much as they are helping me! A good support group goes a very long way!

Breastfeeding support comes in many forms in this digital age. A great resource is Lara Audelo's book, *The Virtual Breastfeeding Culture*. For details on how to contact online and in-person breastfeeding support organizations, see the Resources section.

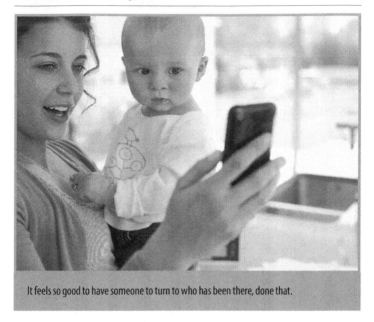

It feels so good to have someone to turn to who has been there, done that.

Changing Your Mind

Every other section of this book assumes that you will follow through on your plans to return to work, and in many families, that is a given. In 2010, almost 41% of the babies born in the U.S. were born to single mothers (CDC, 2013). And in 2013, women were the sole or primary breadwinner in 40% of U.S. households (Wang, Parker, & Taylor, 2013).

However, in some cases, women who fully intended to go back to work after the birth of their baby don't. And sometimes those who think they'll be going back to work full-time find another path. Jennifer E. from

California, USA, a registered nurse, thought at first that she would be her family's sole wage-earner after her baby's birth, but then things changed.

My husband and I always knew one of us was going to stay home with our daughter, even before we got pregnant. My husband had not found steady work in construction and I had a great job as a registered nurse at a prominent health care organization in San Diego. After becoming pregnant, I had an immense desire to move back to our home town, 5 hours north of San Diego. Because my husband couldn't find a job that justified the move, I had to find a job that allowed us to move.

It only took a week to get the new job, and I was four months pregnant already. I worked for this physician for four months, the whole time reassuring them that I was definitely coming back to work after my four-month maternity leave. I was confident that I would have no problem leaving the baby with my husband, and he would have both of our mothers around just in case he needed extra help those first few weeks.

After my daughter was born, there was a lot of tension in the house regarding our agreed arrangement. Figuring out when to pump, how to get the baby to take a bottle, and when to introduce the bottle were all issues I thought about regularly. My husband started to feel uneasy about staying home with the baby, and we constantly looked for jobs for him so that I might be able to stay home. I knew I ultimately always wanted to be the one to stay home with our children, but because the job market wasn't great for construction, I knew I was going to have to make do.

Then I went to work. My daughter was 3 months old, and I was only going to have to go to work for two days then I would have a long weekend before starting my normal schedule. The whole time I was at work, I couldn't enjoy myself. I could do my job, but it was difficult to be happy, and I think it showed. My husband started considering joining the military in order to provide for us. He was willing to be deployed in order to provide for our family. I wasn't very comfortable with that idea, but it was a relief of sorts for both of us to admit that we wanted to switch places. Up until this time we had acted so confident in our plan, but we were fooling ourselves.

I felt so much better going to work knowing I wouldn't have to go much longer. Ultimately I was fired the day I gave notice at work, and I was so glad I didn't have to go through with the rest of my work schedule. We scrambled to get my husband a job, because the military process was long and we had just got it started. He worked for my father doing farm labor for months, and in the end we decided the military would separate us too much for it to be worth it.

Within four months, my husband had three job offers in his chosen field. Ultimately, it has worked out perfectly for us, and we are so satisfied and happy with our choice. The dynamic between us was instantly better when we switched roles, and we have never questioned our current situation, even though I would have been making a lot more money than my husband.

Kim S. from Virginia, USA served full-time in the U.S. Navy after her first child was born, but made a different choice after she had her second baby.

It's not that I didn't want to stop working sooner. I had to wait until the end of my Navy contract. My mother was watching my son so it wasn't dissatisfaction with daycare. I just wanted to spend time with him. When I was ready for a second baby, that's when I dropped my paperwork. The daycare possibility made me nervous. And since I breastfeed, it has been wonderful to not have to worry much about pumping and bottles.

Elizabeth J from North Carolina, USA was 40 with a full-time job as a crisis-line coordinator and counselor at a local domestic-violence agency when she found out she was pregnant. During her pregnancy, she went through an identity crisis and realized she needed to quit her full-time job and eventually started her own part-time business.

It took me almost the entire nine months of my pregnancy to realize that quitting my job was the right thing to do. I'm an intensely loyal person and I loved my work. But the agency was going through a merger and the powers-that-be couldn't tell me what my job would be post-merger. Also, my job was more than full time and to say that it was a huge emotional life suck is an understatement. I gave six-weeks' notice. My last day was 1 month before I was due.

My work has always been important to me, and I couldn't conceive of wanting to be home with our daughter full time. So my plan after leaving my position was to start looking for a full-time job in an alternate field. I was ready to go to an interview when it hit me that I was going to interview for jobs that I didn't care that much about, just because it was decent pay and also because it felt like something that I "should" do. This "should" was grounded in my past identify as someone who works as a professional. When I realized that, I cancelled that interview and called off that search.

I reached out instead to a mentor and said I was looking for very part-time work in any field. She hooked me up with someone looking for help staffing a new upscale shoe boutique. It sounded like a good fit: close by, flexible, pay almost what I was paid in my old job (seriously) and best of all, it wasn't emotionally taxing. I took the job.

At the same time I learned about postpartum doulas and decided it was the path for me. I have always worked supporting women and this seemed another way that just made sense. Over the next year, I started to make sense of my new identity as a person who is someone's mother but still "me."

It became about more than wanting to offer support and help, I realized that we moms need to give ourselves permission to count again. I needed to. We're still important as individuals with needs, even if we are someone's mom. And so a metamorphosis from "just" postpartum doula services to what is now the new business I'm about to launch, where I help new and expecting moms start good habits early by making their needs as important as their partners', babies' or other kids.'

Your Baby's Responses

It's not just mothers who sometimes have strong feelings about their return to work. Depending on temperament, babies sometimes do too. Don't be surprised if your baby begins waking more at night, breastfeeds more often, or is fussier than usual soon after you start work. If this happens, think about how you would like to be treated during a major life change.

If a baby's sleep or feeding pattern changes, some of the mothers I've helped have been told by well-meaning friends, relatives and even health care providers to just let their babies cry. A kinder, gentler strategy during any stressful time is to give your baby extra holding, skin-to-skin contact, and reassurance. Kimberly P. from Texas, USA, a full-time teacher, found that after she started work, her son fed more often after she got home.

> My son was 4.5 months old when I went back to the classroom and he was resilient. It didn't seem to bother him to be away from me much of the day. He enjoyed his caregiver, played with the other children, and never cried when I left him or picked him up. He nursed more frequently at night and on the weekends, and he had his share of colds, but he was (and is) a happy, well-adjusted little guy.

Rachel F. from Kentucky, USA, a full-time public-health counselor, returned to work when her daughters were 12 weeks old. When she started back to work with her second daughter, her baby's feeding patterns changed drastically.

> My first daughter adjusted well to daycare. With my second daughter, my husband was working from home, but she didn't adjust as well to being separated from me. She wouldn't take a bottle during the day and essentially only drank 1 to 1.5 oz. (30 to 45 mL) of breast milk the whole time I was away until my husband introduced a sippy cup to her at 5 months of age. She did much better with that than the bottle. She also reverse cycled most feeds at night when I returned to work, waking up four to six times each night, so on top of feeling sad to be away from her, I was also exhausted each and every day.

Michelle F. from British Columbia, Canada, a full-time registered nurse, returned to work when her son was 15 months old. He showed some signs of stress through unusual bouts of fussiness, which she responded to with love and affection.

> He adapted well to the babysitter. After two weeks of crying when I left, he stopped and welcomed her with open arms. There were times when he was

unexplainably fussy or in need of extra love and affection, which my husband and I doled out happily.

The next chapter focuses on your return to work, with a focus on how to tailor your daily routine to keep your milk production steady, and approaches to night feedings that can help you get more rest.

Keeping Milk Production Stable

This chapter describes what you need to know after returning to work to meet your long-term breastfeeding goals. It explains which of the many day-to-day details are key and which you can ignore. And it explains how your baby's sleep patterns—a hot topic for any parent—can affect the big picture. Knowledge is power, and hopefully the information here will help you make decisions with confidence.

A Vulnerable Time

When you make plans for your first month at work, consider this a vulnerable time, especially if you have a small baby. As you begin working, be very kind to yourself. One study found that mothers who returned to work when their babies were younger than 6 months were more than twice as likely to stop breastfeeding during their first month back compared with mothers not yet on the job (Kimbro, 2006).

In an earlier section, I described strategies for easing this transition. But even if you use all of those tips, this major change won't necessarily be easy. Just like after giving birth, this is a good time to take advantage of all offers of help, keep your focus on what's important, and simplify your life as much as possible.

Wendy R. from Texas, USA returned to work full-time at 7 weeks and learned from that experience.

> I didn't have all the knowledge that I do now ... I would encourage moms to try their best to take off as long as possible from work. This time is precious and you never get it back. If working is an absolute must, then be careful to de-stress your life in every other way possible. Working outside the home and being a new mom and pumping is crazy enough all in itself without adding every other facet of life. Slow down.

Eat Well

One way to take care of yourself is to avoid skipping meals and eat healthy foods. Unless it's extreme, your diet is unlikely to affect how much milk you make or its quality But eating healthy helps keep up your energy and your resistance to illness during this busy time.

Some mothers wonder what to eat when their work meal breaks are spent pumping. But if you're trying to pump one-handed, here are some ideas of healthy foods you can eat with one hand while you pump.

- Your favorite sandwich
- Hard-boiled eggs with a handful of cherry tomatoes
- Slices of turkey rolled-up with a handful of grapes
- A rice cake with cheese spread

Many more practical and nutritious finger foods are listed in the "Making It Work for Moms" brochure at: _http://www.breastfeedingpartners.org/images/pdf/ForMomsFINAL.pdf_:

Understand Basic Dynamics

Worry about milk production is the single biggest concern breastfeeding mothers mention. But being employed and breastfeeding can elevate this from a concern to an obsession. Plus, it doesn't help if you find yourself being regaled with stories of employed mothers who failed to keep their milk flowing.

To meet your goals, you need to understand the basic dynamics of milk production. But more than that, you need to know the impact of your daily routine on these dynamics. I hope my "magic number" concept will remove some of the mystery around milk supply and help you keep your focus on the big picture as you sort out the details (Mohrbacher, 2011).

The Magic Number

Every breastfeeding mother has a magic number. Your magic number is the number of daily milk removals (breastfeeds plus pumps) needed to keep your supply steady over time. To estimate your magic number, think about how many times during the last week or two of your maternity leave that your baby breastfed each day. This may be close to your magic number if all of the following are true:

- Your maternity leave was at least six weeks long.

- You breastfed on cue rather than on a fixed schedule.

- Your exclusively breastfed baby gained weight well.

After returning to work, the key to keeping your milk production steady over the long term is for your number of daily milk removals to stay at or above your magic number. To understand this better, here's a quick review of the two main milk-production dynamics.

Breast Fullness and Milk Production

Breast fullness determines how fast or slow you make milk. "Drained breasts make milk faster and full breasts make milk slower" describes this dynamic. The fuller your breasts become, the slower you make milk. The opposite is also true. Milk production speeds when your breasts are drained more fully. At an average breastfeeding, your baby takes about two-thirds of your milk and leaves one-third. To increase your milk supply as needed, your baby feeds more often and for a longer time, taking a larger percentage of your available milk. This happens naturally when you're with your baby and feeding on cue. You don't even need to think about it. Just let nature take its course.

When you return to work, however, if your baby no longer has access to your breasts around the clock, this means you need to start paying attention. Your milk supply is no longer naturally regulated by your baby.

Why Magic Numbers Vary

Mothers have different magic numbers in part because they have different breast storage capacities. Breast storage capacity refers to the amount of milk available in your breasts when they're at their fullest time of the day. Storage capacity is not about breast size, which is determined mostly by the amount of fatty tissue in your breasts. It is based on the amount of room within your milk-making glands. Smaller-breasted mothers can have a large capacity and larger-breasted mothers can have a small capacity.

Differences in storage capacity account for much of the variations among breastfed babies' feeding patterns:

- Whether your baby usually takes one breast or both.

- Number of daily feedings needed for your baby to gain weight.

- Your baby's longest sleep stretch.

Both large-capacity and small-capacity mothers produce plenty of milk. But their babies feed differently to get the milk they need.

A mother with a large storage capacity has more room in her breasts, so it takes more milk (and more time) for the pressure in her full breasts to build to the point that milk production slows. With more milk available, her baby may always be satisfied with one breast. As he gets older, he may gain weight well with fewer feedings per day than the average baby. And, he may sleep for longer stretches at night than most babies without milk production slowing. The magic number of the mother with a large storage capacity is likely to be lower—maybe only five or six milk removals per day—than the magic number of the mother with a medium or small breast storage capacity.

The mother with a small storage capacity has less milk available at each feeding. Her baby may want both breasts more often, need more daily feedings to get the same amount of milk, and wake more often at night to feed, even as he gets older. Because she has less room for milk in her breasts, they will get full enough for milk production to slow sooner than the mother with a medium or large capacity. If the baby of the small-capacity mother sleeps too long, his mother's breasts quickly become so full of milk that her production slows. A small-capacity mother's magic number will likely be higher—maybe eight or nine milk removals per day—than the mother with a medium or large storage capacity. (The magic number of the average mother is around seven or eight milk removals per day.)

For an idea of where you might fall on the breast-storage-capacity spectrum, see Table 1, which lists several signs that provide clues. You may find it helpful to have a general idea of your magic number, so that you have a starting point from which to plan your daily routine after you return to work.

How to Use Your Magic Number

Your magic number can help you establish a routine that keeps your milk supply steady over the long haul. Rather than basing your schedule on averages or on someone else's experience (whose magic number may be very different from yours), you can tailor your plan to your own body's response.

Because you'll be starting back to work with only an estimate of your magic number, expect that you might need to make adjustments over time. If your estimate is low and your milk production begins to drop, for example, count how many times each 24 hours you're removing milk from your breasts (breast-feeds plus pumps). Your dip in supply tells you that either your number of milk removals is below your magic number or there's an issue with how effectively your pump or your baby is removing your milk. (For example, a baby with a head cold or an ear infection may have trouble nursing for a short time.)

If you've fallen below your magic number, you can reverse this trend by increasing your number of daily milk removals. The sooner you add more milk removals, the sooner you should see improvement. Staying at your magic number should hold your milk production steady. Boosting your daily milk removals above your magic number should increase your supply. Your body's response will tell you what you need to know.

Impact of Daily Routines

Your daily routine can make a big difference in your long-term milk production. During the years I helped employed mothers by phone, I began to notice a pattern.

Role of Breastfeeding

Many of the mothers I spoke with who had dropping milk supplies were pumping the recommended number of times at work, but as the months passed, they breastfed fewer and fewer times at home. Many of these women working full-time, for example, were pumping two-to-three times at work but were only breastfeeding two or three times at home. Some were down to four-to-six total milk removals per day from an average of seven or eight when they were on leave. Most often it was the decrease in breastfeeding that caused them to slip below their magic number and their milk production to slow.

Why did this happen? Many of these mothers were applying bottle-feeding norms to a breastfeeding baby. Many were told that as their babies grew bigger and heavier, they should feed fewer times per day, so they began cutting back. This is common with many bottle-feeding babies, who may consume as much as 7 or 8 oz. (210-240 mL) per feeding. Breastfeeding patterns differ greatly from bottle-feeding patterns. Science tells us that in breastfed babies between 1 and 6 months of age, the volume of milk per feeding and the number of feedings per day doesn't vary by much (Kent et al., 2013). We also know that in part because of these differences, breastfed babies are more likely to have healthier eating habits and weight, while bottle-fed babies are at increased risk of overweight and obesity (Li, Magadia, Fein, & Grummer-Strawn, 2012).

What happens when a breastfeeding mother tries to adopt a bottle-feeding pattern? If her breast storage capacity isn't large enough to sustain it, over time it may cause a decrease in milk production that can lead to slow weight gain or the need to use more and more formula as her pump sessions yield less and less milk. Margarita's experience is a good example of this.

Margarita called me because she was in a quandary. She had been breastfeeding her daughter Luisa for six months, but had been struggling with her milk production since she was 3 months old. Luisa was a sleepy baby from the start and had slept long 10-to-12-hour stretches at night. At first, she breastfed 8-to-10 times per day, and Margarita knew this was normal for a newborn.

But Margarita heard that she should cut back on feedings as Luisa got older. So when she started work at two months, she began to breastfeed less. Almost immediately, her milk production dropped. She started getting up at night to pump because she didn't want to wake her sleeping baby For a month, she gave her this extra milk during the day and was able to continue to exclusively breastfeed. But as she dropped more feedings, she also dropped the nightly pumping. By 4 months, Margarita was pumping twice at work and breastfeeding three times at home. Her daily total was now five milk removals per day, down from 8 to 10 when she was home. Luisa needed more milk than she could pump at work, so she began giving her formula as well.

Margarita tried some of the milk-increasing tips she had heard about. For a while, she took three capsules of the herb fenugreek three times per day, and later her doctor prescribed metoclopramide, a drug that increases milk production in some women. When she did this, her milk production would increase. But when she stopped, her production slowed again.

I explained to Margarita how breast fullness and milk storage capacity affect milk production, and she realized that she had a medium storage capacity. She also now understood what was going wrong. Her strategy of dropping feedings as Luisa grew older was working against her.

She had a breastfeeding goal of one year, and she still wanted to achieve it. What did she do? She increased her number of breastfeeding sessions at home and pumping sessions at work and started pumping right before she went to bed. (She could have done "dream feeds" with Luisa at night—nursing her while she was still half-asleep—but she decided she'd rather pump.) Meeting her breastfeeding goal was important to her, and now that she knew how to reach it, she adjusted her routine to make it happen.

More Breastfeeding Means Less Pumping

Another important dynamic to keep in mind is that that cutting back on breastfeeding at home means your baby will need more expressed milk while you're at work, which you have to work harder to pump. Your baby needs on average about 30 oz. (900 mL) of milk per day. The more milk your

> "...cutting back on breast-feeding at home means your baby will need more expressed milk while you're at work..."

baby gets directly from you, the less milk you need to express. And anything that cuts down on your need to pump is a good thing.

The opposite is true too. The less milk your baby gets from the breast, the more milk you'll need to leave for her while you're at work. What's important to a baby is not how much milk she gets at each feeding, but how much milk she gets over the 24-hour day.

Another way to look at this is that breastfed babies average 3 to 4 oz. (90-120 mL) per feeding. For every breastfeeding you drop, your baby needs another 3 to 4 oz. (90-120 mL) while you're at work.

Ways to Fit in More Breastfeeding

After you return to work, what can you do to encourage more breastfeeding? You have several options.

- **Cluster feedings together before you leave for work.** If you leave in the morning, breastfeed twice: once when you wake up and again right before you leave your baby. (If your baby is asleep, wake her to feed, or do a "dream feed," so she is full when you leave.)

- **Consider nursing midday.** Can you go to your baby for one or more feedings during your work day or have your baby brought to you for breast-feeding?

- **Breastfeed as soon as you and your baby are reunited after work.** If she seems hungry just before you arrive, suggest the caregiver give as little milk as possible until you get there.

- **Cluster feedings together when you're home after work.**

- **Nurse before your bedtime.** If your baby goes to sleep for the night earlier than you, do a "dream feed" right before you go to bed, and if your baby sleeps for very long stretches at night, do another you if you awaken during the night.

Babies can be coaxed to "dream feed" when they're in a light sleep, which you can recognize because you'll see movement, such as eyes moving under eyelids. If you lean back and lay your lightly sleeping baby on top of you, this will trigger her feeding reflexes, and she may start to root. Amazingly, babies don't have to be awake to breastfeed effectively.

Your Pump Schedule and Your Magic Number

Many mothers assume when they go back to work that they need to pump the same number of times or the same time of day that they had been breastfeeding at home. That's not actually necessary. To keep your milk production steady, plan to stay at or above your magic number. But the exact times you pump or breastfeed are not crucial. If possible, try to avoid going longer than seven or eight hours between milk removals (full breasts make milk slower), but other than that, you have the freedom to structure your day in the way that makes most sense for your unique situation.

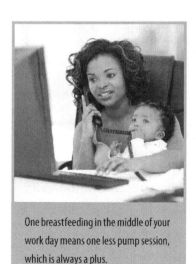

One breastfeeding in the middle of your work day means one less pump session, which is always a plus.

Your breastfeeding pattern also plays a role. Nora C. from Ontario, Canada shared her experience after she started work full-time: "I returned to work when my son was just under 6 months. He wouldn't take pumped milk at all during the day, so I just breastfed about five or six times before I went to bed (4 pm, 5 pm, 6 pm, 7-8 pm, and 10:30 pm or so) and twice in the morning before work (5:30 am and 7:15 am)."

Table 2: Breastfeeding Patterns

Breastfeeding Times	Longest Stretches	Comments
5:30 a.m. 7:15 a.m. 4 p.m. 5 p.m. 6 p.m. 7-8 p.m. 10:30 p.m.	7:15 a.m.-4 p.m. (8 hr., 45 min.) 10:30 p.m.-5:30 a.m. (7 hr.)	* Seven breastfeeds/day are enough * But full breasts make milk slower, so Nora should shorten her longest stretch to ≤7 hr. with one mid-work pump or breastfeed

Nora breastfed seven times each day, which—since she had a medium breast storage capacity—would probably be enough to keep her production stable without any pumping at work except for that nearly nine-hour stretch during her work day. To keep her milk supply steady, one option would be to pump once in the middle of her work day so her very full breasts did not make milk slower. Another option was for her caregiver to bring her baby to her to breastfeed (or for Nora to go to her baby) during her longest break.

Your pumping plan should take your magic number into account. How? Plan to pump the minimum number of times at work needed to both provide the milk you'd like to leave for your baby and to maintain your production. If you have a large storage capacity, you will likely pump more milk at a session than other mothers, so that factors into the equation too. If you haven't yet determined your breast storage capacity, review again Table 1 and see where you might fall on this spectrum.

As mentioned before, if you have a very large breast storage capacity, your magic number will probably be five or six. If your baby breastfeeds four times when you're together, this means two pumps at work should be enough to keep milk production stable. (Or you could do five breastfeeds at home and one pump at work.) On the other hand, if you have a small storage capacity, your magic number may be eight or nine. If your baby breastfeeds only four times at home, you would need to pump four or five times at work, which would be impractical for most women. Instead, for most it would make far more sense to breastfeed more at home. By breastfeeding six or seven times each day at home, you would be able to keep your milk flowing well with only two pump sessions at work.

Sleep and Night Feedings

With a clear understanding of how milk production works, you can appreciate why night feedings can be such an important part of meeting your breast-feeding goals.

- The number of milk removals over 24 hours regulates milk production.

- Allowing your breasts to stay too full for too long causes milk production to slow.

- Going for very long stretches without breast-feeding when you're at home makes it more challenging to keep your milk removals at or above your magic number.

- Long stretches without breastfeeding at home also means you need to leave more pumped milk for your baby while you're at work.

What is a "very long stretch?" Going six or seven hours is unusual in a breastfeeding baby, but that is not long enough to cause milk production to slow in most women. However, stretches as long as eight-to-12 hours are a real challenge for many.

The Dilemma

In Western countries, parents feel a strong social pressure for their babies to sleep for long stretches at night. One mother I spoke to shows how this can play out. Tawana was on her maternity leave and was preparing to go back to work soon. Her baby, Clevon, was about 6 weeks old. Like most new mothers, she was often asked how many hours her baby slept at night. Tawana discovered that if she put Clevon in a swing, as long as it kept moving, he would stay asleep the entire night (sleeping in a swing is not recommended for safety reasons). But Tawana didn't want to put the swing in her bedroom, because its noise would keep her partner awake. And she didn't want to leave her baby alone while in motion all night in the swing. When I spoke to her, she was sleeping on the sofa in the living room next to her baby's swing and getting up every hour to check on him. Clevon's weight gain had slowed during the week or two he had spent his nights in the swing.

After asking Tawana some questions, it seemed clear that she had a small-to-medium breast storage capacity and such long stretches between milk removals had reduced her milk supply, causing the slowed weight gain. Also, she was exhausted from getting up every hour all night. When Tawana realized that using the swing to keep her baby asleep longer was the root cause of both her exhaustion and her milk-production issues, she decided it made more sense for her baby to sleep in her room and to breastfeed at night again. In her case, her baby's long sleep stretch had led to problems, and she decided to stop making his uninterrupted sleep her top priority.

Many mothers hope their baby will "sleep through the night" during the early months. It is not unusual for some breastfed babies (even newborns) to have one four-to-five-hour sleep stretch, and that is fine. But if your baby sleeps longer than about seven hours and your breast storage capacity is small or medium, as Tawana found, it can lead to milk production issues. This is not something you normally need to worry about while you're on leave, because if milk production slows, your baby naturally breastfeeds more often to boost it again. But in Tawana's case, the moving swing had blunted her baby's natural feeding cues. One of the risks of overusing devices like swings and pacifiers is that they can delay and even eliminate some feedings, which can lower milk production.

There is a natural tension between the Western cultural pressure to encourage babies to sleep for long stretches at night and the importance of frequent milk removal to milk production. Continuing regular night feedings may be important to reaching your breastfeeding target. Yet no one questions the fact that you also need your rest, especially when you're expected to be productive at your job. How do you reconcile these seemingly opposite needs?

Getting the Rest You Need

Fatigue is a normal part of new parenthood, no matter how a baby is fed. During your leave, one way to make up for lost sleep is to sleep when your baby sleeps. That's not possible, though, once you're back at work. So what do you do? First, let's look at two common misconceptions.

Giving formula or bottles at night may actually mean less sleep. It may seem logical that you would get more sleep if you feed your baby formula before bed or if someone else handles some of the night feedings. But research found that mothers who breastfeed around the clock get between 25 and 45 more minutes of sleep, spend more time in deeper sleep, and feel less tired than mixed-feeding or formula-feeding mothers (Blyton, Sullivan, & Edwards, 2002; Doan, Gardiner, Gay, & Lee, 2007; Kendall-Tackett, Cong, & Hale, 2011).

Although babies fed formula do seem to sleep more, their mothers don't. The Doan study suggested this is because mothers' sleep is disrupted when others handle night feedings. The Kendall-Tackett study found that the breastfeeding mothers reported more total sleep time and took less time to get back to sleep. In the Blyton study, sleep researchers analyzed the brain waves of women during sleep and found that exclusively breastfeeding mothers spent more time in deeper sleep than exclusively formula-feeding mothers and women without infants. It may be that the hormones released during breastfeeding improve sleep quality and the more you breastfeed, the better you sleep.

Solid foods don't increase a baby's sleep time. The popular belief that solid foods will help babies sleep longer actually has no basis in fact. In one study, about the same number of babies began sleeping more at night whether they received solid foods or not (Macknin, Medendorp, & Maier, 1989). Sleeping longer at night is a developmental milestone that is unrelated to solid foods.

So if giving formula and solids won't mean more sleep, what *can* you do?

Keep your baby nearby at night. Keeping your baby close is key. The less you have to move around at night to breastfeed, the easier it is to get back to sleep. This can also be a lifesaver for your baby. The American Academy of Pediatrics recommends that babies sleep in their parents' room for the first 6 months to prevent SIDS (American Academy of Pediatrics, 2011).

There are many safe-sleep options. Every family develops its own nighttime variations that work best for them. Here are some choices.

- Your baby sleeps in a bassinet next to your bed.

- Your baby sleeps in a sidecar bed attached to yours.

- Your baby sleeps in a crib with the side next to your bed removed and the crib pushed against your bed for easy access.

- Your baby sleeps in a crib elsewhere in your room.

- Your baby sleeps in your bed (using the safe sleep guidelines below) for all or part of the night.

- Your baby (or you and your baby together) sleep on a mattress (or a pallet, a sleeping bag, etc.) on the floor in your room.

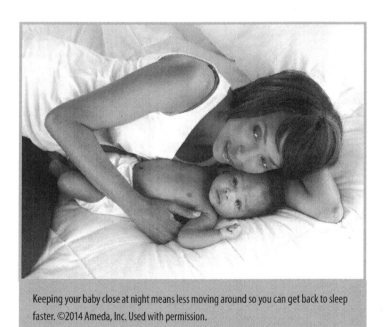

Keeping your baby close at night means less moving around so you can get back to sleep faster. ©2014 Ameda, Inc. Used with permission.

Wherever your baby sleeps, you need to know about safe and unsafe sleeping practices. Those listed below are adapted from the guidelines of the Academy of Breastfeeding Medicine (*www.bfmed.org*). The American Academy of Pediatrics also published safe-sleep recommendations (American Academy of Pediatrics, 2011).

If you sleep in a standard American adult bed, products are available, such as guard rails and bolsters, that can prevent falls and make your bed safe for your baby. Or you can put your mattress on the floor away from walls. In Japan, where bedsharing is the norm and many families sleep on futons on the floor, their SIDS rate is among the lowest in the world (McKenna & McDade, 2005). Dawn B. from Georgia, USA, who worked full time in customer service for a manufacturing company, found regular bedsharing the best answer for her and her family.

> My baby was 10 weeks old when I returned to work. I truly believe that bedsharing helped me continue breastfeeding while working. I've described having a baby and working as holding down three full-time jobs: the baby, your job, and your household/relationship with your partner. Anything that makes that easier is a plus. Getting sleep at night makes it easier.

Most parents sleep with their baby some of the time, sometimes unintentionally, so as a precaution, make your bed safe for your baby. Even if you don't plan for you and your baby to fall asleep there, breastfeeding releases hormones that relax you, so it may happen.

Learn to breastfeed lying down. No mother should have to choose between getting her rest and feeding her baby. Breastfeeding lying down allows you to sleep and feed at the same time. Even if this doesn't come easily to you, know that it gets easier with practice.

Safe Sleeping Practices for any Location

- Put your baby on his back to sleep.
- Use a firm, flat surface, such as a firm mattress on the floor away from walls, or a co-sleeping baby bed (sidecar) or crib that can attach to an adult bed.
- Tuck in any blankets around the mattress to avoid covering your baby's head.
- Dress your baby in a warm sleeper if the room is cold.
- Keep your baby in your room at night for the first six months.

Practice this at a time you feel awake and alert. Your own best way of breastfeeding lying down may be unique and will depend on your body type. See the images below for some approaches to try.

Unsafe sleeping practices

- Your baby should not bedshare with a smoker.
- Don't sleep with your baby on a sofa, couch, recliner, daybed, or waterbed, or with pillows, stuffed toys, or loose bedding near baby.
- Don't bedshare if impaired by alcohol, sedatives, or other drugs.
- Don't sleep in a bed with an adjacent space where your baby could fall or that could trap your baby.

Nap on your day off. Even if you can't fit in catnaps on work days, getting in a good nap on at least one day off can make all the difference. Kristine R. from Connecticut, USA, a full-time middle-school teacher considered this strategy a lifesaver.

I went back when my kids were 8.5 and 11 months. They woke several times a night up to about 23 months. I did many things to keep supply high and satisfy my baby's need for closeness (cluster-feed before and after work, nurse a lot on the weekends, nurse at night, bedsharing), but almost every weekend, I got in a good nap on one of the days. That was key for me: catching up on sleep when someone else could be in charge of the baby! I made sure to not over plan for the weekends so I could be sure to catch a nap. That was something I found easy to do because after a busy week of being a working parent, I just wanted to relax and be with my kids anyway. Taking an hour or 2 to myself to nap made me able to give more of myself at night and during the week, which were pretty demanding.

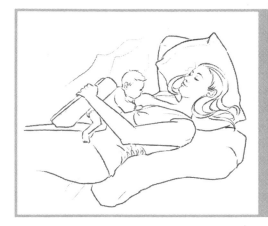

The baby's head rests on the bed and the mother leans back into the pillow. Notice the rolled baby blanket the mother wedged behind her baby leaves her head free to angle back.

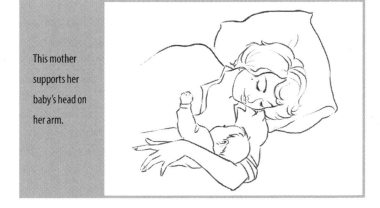

This mother supports her baby's head on her arm.

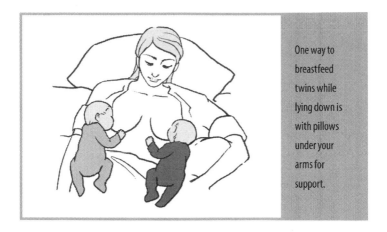

One way to breastfeed twins while lying down is with pillows under your arms for support.

What to Expect as Your Baby Grows

Although you can expect for your baby's sleep patterns to change as he grows, keep your expectations realistic. On average, breastfed babies wake as much at night to feed at 6 months as they do at 1 month (Kent et al., 2006). Even into their second year, breastfeeding babies and toddlers do not have the same sleep patterns as non-breastfed babies.

But individual differences play a role in babies' sleep too. Differences in mothers' breast storage capacity, for example, mean that some thriving breastfed babies sleep for long stretches at night early on, while others need to breastfeed at night even at 8 months, 10 months, and beyond. Many mothers expect that as their babies grow, they will sleep more and more. However, even the baby who has been sleeping well at night for a while often starts waking again as the discomfort of teething begins. More frequent night waking can also happen as babies begin learning new skills, such as crawling and walking. So if your baby starts sleeping for long periods at night, don't expect this will continue. There are many reasons babies wake at night and want comfort, even when they're not hungry. You may find that as your baby grows, your nighttime solutions change. That's what happened with Kaia and her daughter.

> My solution was various forms of co-sleeping. She slept in her swing in our room for months because of severe reflux. I tried bedsharing then but she couldn't because it was too flat. At age 10 months or so, she was more comfortable lying flat so I moved her to our bed. When she started being really mobile in her sleep, I converted her crib into a side-car because of fears she'd roll out of the bed. We did that for a few months until my husband went away for work for a long period. We moved her crib to the corner of our room with the plan being to transition her, but I enjoyed having her back in bed with me, so I just bedshared. She is now 2, nurses only to sleep in our bed, and then is put into her crib in our room asleep. If she wakes during the night and will not go back to sleep, she comes into our bed with us. She woke every two hours until she was over a year old, so I don't know how I would've managed without co-sleeping in its various permutations.

Every family decides how to best handle their babies' night feedings. Be open to trying different strategies at different ages. As Kaia and her family found, both her and her baby's needs and preferences changed as the months passed.

Now that we've covered the basics on how to plan your day (and night) to ensure good milk production, let's address how to know and what to do if your milk production needs a boost.

5

Sample Plans for Different Work Schedules

There are many ways to plan your day. The following sample plans are intended to give you some ideas to try or to suggest to your employer. Ultimately, as always, do what works best for you.

Full-Time Job

A full-time job may consist of the traditional eight-hour day, five days per week. But it may not. Some women work much longer days, so samples of both are shown here. These schedules should work well for women with a small to medium breast storage capacity. If you have a large storage capacity, you may be able to pump fewer times during your work day without a dip in your milk production.

Eight-Hour Workdays

Traditional 8 a.m. to 5 p.m. work day, small-to-medium storage capacity

- 5:30 a.m.: Wake, nurse baby (dream feed), get ready for the day.

- 7:15 a.m.: Breastfeed baby at childcare provider before leaving for work.

- 8:00 a.m.: Arrive at work.

- 10:00-10:25 a.m.: Pump (with a drink and/or snack).

- 12:00-1:00 p.m.: Lunch break, pump or breast-feed while eating.

- 3:00-3:25 p.m.: Pump (with a drink and/or snack).

- 5:00 p.m.: Leave work.

- 5:20 p.m.: Breastfeed at caregiver before leaving for home.

- At home: Encourage frequent feedings.

Job with afternoon/evening shift, small-to-medium storage capacity

- During the morning: Encourage frequent feedings.

- 12:15 p.m.: Feed baby at childcare provider right before leaving for work.

- 1:00 p.m.: Arrive at work.

- 3:00 3:25 p.m.: Pump break (with a drink and/ or snack).

- 6:00-6:30 p.m.: Meal break, pump or breastfeed while eating.

- 8:30-8:55 p.m.: Pump break (with a drink and/ or snack).

- 10:00 p.m.: Leave work.

- 10:20 p.m.: Do a dream feed with baby at child-care provider before leaving for home.

- At home: Encourage frequent feedings.

12-Hour Workdays

Day job, small-to-medium storage capacity

- 5:30 a.m.: Wake, nurse baby (dream feed), get ready for the day.

- 7:15 a.m.: Breastfeed baby at childcare provider before leaving for work.

- 8:00 a.m.: Arrive at work.

- 10:00-10:25 a.m.: Pump (with a drink and/or snack).

- 12:00-1:00 p.m.: Lunch break, pump or breast-feed while eating.

- 3:00-3:25 p.m.: Pump (with a drink and/or snack).

- 6:00-6:30 p.m.: Dinner break, pump or breast-feed while eating.

- 8:00 p.m.: Leave for childcare provider.

- 8:30 p.m.: Breastfeed at caregiver before leaving for home.

- At home: Encourage frequent feedings.

Part-Time Job

Your need to pump will vary, depending on your job schedule. For example, if you'll be working three days per week, milk production may be easier to manage if you alternate days at work with days at home. That way, if your daily total dips one day, your baby can nurse like crazy the next day so that it rebounds. Choose a schedule that works best for you. Here are some possibilities.

Several Long Days

See the 8-hour and 12-hour sample schedules in the previous section as a starting point. If you have a large breast storage capacity or you are alternating work days, you may be able to keep your milk stable with fewer pump sessions per day.

Many Short Days

To pump or not to pump, that is the question. The length of your work day and your breast storage capacity will determine the best plan for you. If your work day is no longer than the longest stretch between feedings at home, then pumping at work is optional. If you want to store milk for work days, you can pump after feedings at home. Here's an example. Swati returned to work as a barrista in a coffee shop when her baby, Taj, was 8 weeks old. She was scheduled for five six-hour shifts per week, from 12 to 6 p.m. During her maternity leave, Taj had begun sleeping for six-hour stretches at night. When he woke to feed, Swati felt full but not uncomfortable. Taj took a 4 oz. (160 mL) bottle while she was at work. To store milk for her baby, rather than pumping in the middle of her work shift, Swati decided to pump once every morning about an hour after her first feeding and again after work after she nursed Taj. During those pump sessions, she was able to store enough milk for the one feeding her baby took during work.

But going for six-hour stretches without pumping or breastfeeding wouldn't be the best option for every mother. Here's another example. Breastfeeding was going well for Hiroko and her baby Sen. Hiroko returned to work as a server in a catering business when Sen was 12 weeks old. She worked evenings at events, and her shifts were six hours long. During his first three months, Sen had never gone longer than four hours between feedings and when he did, Hiroko felt full-to-bursting. Hiroko arranged to take pumping breaks midway in her shift, at about the three-hour mark, at which she pumped enough for her baby's feeding on her next work day.

6

Resources

Finding Skilled Breastfeeding Help

If you're in need of breastfeeding help, don't wait to find someone. Usually, the sooner you get help, the easier it is to solve your problem. When contacting local breastfeeding specialists, be aware that different credentials reflect different levels of education and training. A variety of initials (CLC, CLE, CBE, CBC, LE, and others) are awarded after attending a brief training course, usually less than one week long. A person with these initials may be able to provide some help but may have limited skills, understanding, and experience.

The credential IBCLC, however, indicates—at the least—a basic competence in the field of lactation. These initials stand for "International Board Certified Lactation Consultant." To receive this credential, a person must pass an all-day certifying exam. To qualify to take that exam, she must first have a combi-nation of formal education, breastfeeding education, and thousands of hours working one-on-one with breastfeeding mothers and babies. There are several ways you can find a local IBCLC.

- Click on the "Find a Lactation Consultant" link on _www.ilca.org_ and enter your ZIP or postal code. ILCA is the International Lactation Consultant Association, the professional association for lactation consultants. Not all international board certified lactation consultants are members.

- Contact your local birthing facility and ask to speak to the breastfeeding specialist. Ask if she can help you or if she knows someone in your community who can.

- Contact your local public-health department and ask if there is any IBCLCs on staff who can help you.

- Contact mother-to-mother breastfeeding support people in your area (see next section) and ask them for suggestions. They may know the best choices in your area.

Another possible source of skilled breastfeeding help is the mother-to-mother support organizations listed in the next section. These experienced breast-feeding mothers work as volunteers to help other mothers. Their skill level can run the gamut from highly skilled to inexperienced. Hopefully, if they can't help you, they'll know someone who can.

Getting the Support You Need

Don't underestimate the importance of ongoing breastfeeding support. What's really great today is that breastfeeding support comes in many forms. Even if you are in a remote location, work odd hours, or lack safe, reliable transportation, you can access the many Facebook groups and online forums that support employed breastfeeding mothers. To get a sense of what's out there and its immense value, see Lara Audelo's book, *The Virtual Breastfeeding Culture: Seeking Mother-to-Mother Support in the Digital Age.*

Mother-to-Mother Breastfeeding Organizations

It's always a plus to have choices, and sometimes there's just no substitute for spending face time with other mothers and babies. Mother-to-mother breastfeeding organizations that offer in-person meetings (as well as online and Facebook support options) are:

- Breastfeeding USA (*www.breastfeedingusa.org*), this rapidly growing nonprofit organization was formed in 2010 with a focus on providing evidence-based information and support in a variety of formats.

- Australian Breastfeeding Association (*www.breastfeeding.asn.au*). This long-standing beacon of breastfeeding support offers a range of services, such as classes, email counseling, a 24-hour Breastfeeding Helpline, online forums, and local support groups.

In the U.K., there are several national breastfeeding support organizations. A list of their links is at: *http://www.nhs.uk/Conditions/pregnancy-and-baby/pages/breastfeeding-help-support.aspx#close*

Another mother-to-mother option in most countries is La Leche League International (*www.llli.org*), the grandmother of breastfeeding support, which has been helping mothers since 1956 and offers in-person meetings, phone, and email help. One way La Leche League differs from other breastfeeding organizations is that it requires its leaders to follow its parenting philosophy, which is consistent with attachment parenting. It does not require those who seek help from La Leche League to follow its philosophy.

Doulas

"Doula" comes from the Greek word for servant, and refers to someone who provides practical and emotional help to women before, during, and after birth. Many doulas also offer breastfeeding help and support.

- DONA International (_www.dona.org_) lists labor-support and postpartum doulas.

- Find a Doula, Australia (_http://www.findadoula. com.au/_) to locale doulas in Australia.

- Doula U.K. (_http://doula.org.uk/_) to locate labor and postpartum/postnatal doulas.

Websites

The internet can be an unreliable place. All breast-feeding websites are definitely not created equal! Here are some that you can trust.

- _Kellymom.com_ is a great site that includes articles on almost every aspect of breastfeeding.

- _NancyMohrbacher.com_ includes a section for employed breastfeeding mothers and many articles on hot topics.

- _BreastfeedingMadeSimple.com_ is the companion site for the book I co-authored with Kathleen Kendall-Tackett, _Breastfeeding Made Simple_. It has many resources for a wide range of breast-feeding concerns and common challenges.

- _WomensHealth.gov/breastfeeding/government-in-action/business-case.html_ Here you can download _The Business Case for Breastfeeding_, which includes materials for mothers, human resources, CEOs, etc. A treasure trove of great resources.

- *Womenshealth.gov/breastfeeding/employer-solutions/index.php* A new U.S. Government website for working and breastfeeding mothers and their employers.

- *BestforBabes.org* offers resources for employed mothers, as well as ways to avoid "booby traps."

- *BreastfeedingPartners.org* Click on the "Work & School" tab to find its *Making It Work Toolkit,* a great resource.

- *Workandpump.com* This site is an oldie but a goodie that is chock full of great info.

- *BreastfeedingUSA.org* offers many helpful articles and a locator for local support.

- *Breastfeedinginc.ca* has many helpful articles and videos by Canadian pediatrician and lactation consultant, Dr. Jack Newman.

- *Isisonline.org.uk* offers evidence-based information for parents and professionals about infant sleep norms.

- *Lowmilksupply.org* was created by two lactation consultants who specialize in milk production issues.

Free Online Videos

Hand Expression:

http://newborns.stanford.edu/Breastfeeding/HandExpression.html

Hands-on Pumping:

http://newborns.stanford.edu/Breastfeeding/MaxProduction.html

Paced Bottle Feeding for the Breastfed Baby:

http://www.youtube.com/
watch?v=UH4T7OOSzGs&feature=youtube

Reverse Pressure Softening. How to Relieve Engorgement:

*http://www.youtube.com/watch?v=2_*
RD9HNrOJ8&oref=http%3A%2F%2Fwww.youtube.
com%2Fwatch%3Fv%3D2_RD9HNrOJ8&has_verified=1

Books

These resources would be great additions to any employed mother's bookshelf.

Audelo, L. (2013). *The virtual breastfeeding culture: Seeking mother-to-mother support in the digital age.* Amarillo, TX Praeclarus Press.

Mohrbacher, N., & Kendall-Tackett, K. (2010). *Breastfeeding made simple: Seven natural laws for nursing mothers, 2ⁿᵈ Ed.* Oakland, CA: New Harbinger Publications.

Mohrbacher, N. (2013). *Breastfeeding solutions: Quick tips for the most common nursing challenges.* Oakland, CA: New Harbinger Publications.

Peterson, A., & Harmer, M. (2010). *Balancing breast and bottle: Reaching your breastfeeding goals.* Amarillo, TX: Hale Publishing.

Rapley, G., & Murkett, T. (2010). *Baby-led weaning: The essential guide to introducing solid foods—and helping your baby to grow up a happy and confident eater.* New York: The Experiment.

Roche-Paull, R. (2010). *Breastfeeding in combat boots: A survival guide to successful breastfeeding while serving in the military.* Amarillo, TX: Hale Publishing.

West, D., & Marasco, L. (2009). *The breastfeeding mothers' guide to making more milk.* New York: McGraw-Hill.

Smartphone App

Here's a basic breastfeeding resource you can download to your Android or iPhone. It covers the 30 most common breastfeeding challenges, and includes the milk-storage guidelines in this book. Use your smartphone to open this link and you're on your way.

Breastfeeding Solutions by Nancy Mohrbacher. (2013). Available for Android and iPhones from Amazon, Google Play, and the App Store. *http://www.nancymohrbacher.com/app-support/*

Breast Pumps to Buy or Rent

Here is the contact information for the three recommended breast-pump brands.

Ameda Breast Pumps

To locate an Ameda rental pump or purchase an Ameda Purely Yours pump near you, call Ameda Breastfeeding Products, at 1-866-99AMEDA (1-866-992-6332), or go online to *www.Ameda.com*.

Hygeia Breast Pumps

To locate a Hygeia rental pump or a Hygeia Enjoye purchase pump near you, call Hygeia at 1-888-786-7466 or go online to *www.Hygeiainc.com*.

Medela Breast Pumps

To locate a Medela rental pump or purchase a Medela Pump In Style or Freestyle pump near you, contact Medela, Inc., at 1-800-TELLYOU (in the U.S.) or go online to *www.medela.com*.

Other Products

Hands-Free Pumping Devices

For the latest commercial products that help you pump hands-free, just Google "hands-free pumping." Some women make their own. Here are two options:

- This free tutorial uses elastic hair bands: *http://kellymom.com/bf/pumpingmoms/pumping/hands-free-pumping/*

- This one (be sure to click on the pictures) uses rubber bands: *http://www.workandpump.com/handsfree.htm*

Prevent Milk Leakage

To find LilyPadz, the silicone product that applies pressure to the nipples to prevent milk leakage, go online to *www.lilypadz.com*.

Collect Leaked Milk

To find Milkies milk savers, the container you wear to collect milk while your baby breastfeeds, go online to *http://www.mymilkies.com/milksaver*.

References

American Academy of Pediatrics (AAP). (2012). Breastfeeding and the use of human milk. *Pediatrics, 129*(3), e827-e841.

American Academy of Pediatrics. (AAP). (2011). SIDS and other sleep-related infant deaths: expansion of recommendations for a safe infant sleeping environment. *Pediatrics, 128*(5), 1030-1039.

American Academy of Pediatrics. (AAP). (2001). The use and misuse of fruit juice in pediatrics. *Pediatrics, 107*(5), 1210-1213.

Blyton, D. M., Sullivan, C. E., & Edwards, N. (2002). Lactation is associated with an increase in slow-wave sleep in women. *Journal of Sleep Research, 11*(4), 297-303.

Boushey, H., & Glynn, S. J. (2012). There are significant business costs to replacing employees. Retrieved from: http://www.americanprogress.org/wp-content/uploads/2012/11/CostofTurnover.pdf

Brusseau, R. (1998). *Bacterial analysis of refrigerated human milk following infant feeding. Unpublished senior thesis.* Concordia University.

Centers for Disease Control and Prevention. (CDC). (2013). *Unmarried childbearing.* Retrieved from: http://www.cdc.gov/nchs/fastats/unmarry.htm

Centers for Disease Control and Prevention. (CDC). (2012). *Percentage of breastfed U.S. children who are supplemented with infant formula, by birth year.* Retrieved from http://www.cdc.gov/breastfeeding/data/nis_data/

Chatterji, P., & Markowitz, S. (2012). Family leave after childbirth and the mental health of new mothers. *The Journal of Mental Health Policy and Economics, 15*(2), 61-76.

Cohen, R., Lange, L., & Slusser, W. (2002). A description of a male-focused breastfeeding promotion corporate lactation program. *Journal of Human Lactation, 18*(1), 61-65.

Cohen, R., & Mrtek, M. B. (1994). The impact of two corporate lactation programs on the incidence and duration of breast-feeding by employed mothers. *American Journal of Health Promotion, 8*(6), 436-441.

Cohen, R., Mrtek, M. B., & Mrtek, R. G. (1995). Comparison of maternal absenteeism and infant illness rates among breast-feeding and formula-feeding women in two corporations. *American Journal of Health Promotion, 10*(2), 148-153.

Colson, S. D., Meek, J. H., & Hawdon, J. M. (2008). Optimal positions for the release of primitive neonatal reflexes stimulating breastfeeding. *Early Human Development, 84*(7), 441-449.

DaMota, K., Banuelos, J., Goldbronn, J., Vera-Beccera, L. E., & Heinig, M. J. (2012). Maternal request for in-hospital supplementation of healthy breastfed infants among low-income women. *Journal of Human Lactation, 28*(4), 476-482.

Dewey, K. G., & Brown, K. H. (2003). Update on technical issues concerning complementary feeding of young children in developing countries and implications for intervention programs. *Food and Nutrition Bulletin, 24*(1), 5-28.

Doan, T., Gardiner, A., Gay, C. L., & Lee, K. A. (2007). Breast-feeding increases sleep duration of new parents. *Journal of Perinatal and Neonatal Nursing, 21*(3), 200-206.

Dunn, B. F., Zavela, K. J., Cline, A. D., & Cost, P. A. (2004). Breastfeeding practices in Colorado businesses. *Journal of Human Lactation, 20*(2), 170-177.

Geddes, D. T. (2009). The use of ultrasound to identify milk ejection in women: Tips and pitfalls. *International Breastfeeding Journal, 4*, 5.

Goldblum, R. M., Garza, C., Johnson, C. A., Harrist, R., & Nichols, B. L. (1981). Human milk banking I: Effects of container upon immunologic factors in mature milk. *Nutrition Research, 1*, 449-459.

Hale, T. W. (2012). *Medications & Mothers' Milk* (15th Ed.). Amarillo, TX: Hale Publishing.

Hammond, K. A. (1997). Adaptation of the maternal intestine during lactation. *Journal of Mammary Gland Biology and Neoplasia, 2*(3), 243-252.

Heinig, M. J., Nommsen, L. A., Peerson, J. M., Lonnerdal, B., & Dewey, K. G. (1993). Energy and protein intakes of breast-fed and formula-fed infants during the first year of life and their association with growth velocity: the DARLING Study. *American Journal of Clinical Nutrition, 58*(2), 152-161.

Hennart, P., Delogne-Desnoeck, J., Vis, H., & Robyn, C. (1981). Serum levels of prolactin and milk production in women during a lactation period of thirty months. *Clinical Endocrinology (Oxf), 14*(4), 349-353.

Hicks, J. B. (Ed.). (2006). *Hirikani's daughters: Women who scale modern mountains to combine breastfeeding and working.* Schaumburg, Illinois: La Leche League International.

Hill, P. D., Aldag, J. C., Chatterton, R. T., & Zinaman, M. (2005). Comparison of milk output between mothers of preterm and term infants: The first 6 weeks after birth. *Journal of Human Lactation, 21*(1), 22-30.

HRSA. (2008). *The Business Case for Breastfeeding.* Retrieved from: http://www.womenshealth.gov/breastfeeding/government-in-action/business-case-for-breastfeeding/.

Islam, M. M., Peerson, J. M., Ahmed, T., Dewey, K. G., & Brown, K. H. (2006). Effects of varied energy density of complementary foods on breast-milk intakes and total energy consumption by healthy, breastfed Bangladeshi children. *American Journal of Clinical Nutrition, 83*(4), 851-858.

Jones, E., & Hilton, S. (2009). Correctly fitting breast shields are the key to lactation success for pump dependent mothers following preterm delivery. *Journal of Neonatal Nursing, 15*(1), 14-17.

Jones, F., & Tully, M. R. (2011). *Best practices for expressing, storing and handling human milk* (3rd Ed.). Raleigh, NC: Human Milk Banking Association of North America.

Kearney, M. H., & Cronenwett, L. (1991). Breastfeeding and employment. *Journal of Obstetric, Gynecologic & Neonatal Nursing, 20*(6), 471-480.

Kendall-Tackett, K., Cong, Z., & Hale, T. W. (2011). The effect of feeding method on sleep duration, maternal well-being, and postpartum depression. *Clinical Lactation, 2*(2), 22-26.

Kent, J. C. (2007). How breastfeeding works. *Journal of Midwifery & Women's Health, 52*(6), 564-570.

Kent, J. C., Hepworth, A. R., Sherriff, J. L., Cox, D. B., Mitoulas, L. R., & Hartmann, P. E. (2013). Longitudinal changes in breastfeeding patterns from 1 to 6 months of lactation. *Breastfeeding Medicine, 8*, 401-407.

Kent, J. C., Mitoulas, L., Cox, D. B., Owens, R. A., & Hartmann, P. E. (1999). Breast volume and milk production during extended lactation in women. *Experimental Physiology, 84*(2), 435-447.

Kent, J. C., Mitoulas, L. R., Cregan, M. D., Geddes, D. T., Larsson, M., Doherty, D. A., et al. (2008). Importance of vacuum for breast milk expression. *Breastfeeding Medicine, 3*(1), 11-19.

Kent, J. C., Mitoulas, L. R., Cregan, M. D., Ramsay, D. T., Doherty, D. A., & Hartmann, P. E. (2006). Volume and frequency of breastfeedings and fat content of breast milk throughout the day. *Pediatrics, 117*(3), e387-395.

Kent, J. C., Prime, D. K., & Garbin, C. P. (2011). Principles for maintaining or increasing breast milk production. *Journal of Obstetric, Gynecologic, & Neonatal Nursing.* doi: 10.1111/j.1552-6909.2011.01313.x.

Kent, J. C., Ramsay, D. T., Doherty, D., Larsson, M., & Hartmann, P. E. (2003). Response of breasts to different stimulation patterns of an electric breast pump. *Journal of Human Lactation, 19*(2), 179-186.

Kimbro, R. T. (2006). On-the-job moms: Work and breastfeeding initiation and duration for a sample of low-income women. *Maternal & Child Health Journal, 10*(1), 19-26.

Kline, T. S., & Lash, S. R. (1964). The bleeding nipple of pregnancy and postpartum period: A cytologic and histologic study. *Acta Cytologica, 8,* 336-340.

Kramer, M. S., Guo, T., Platt, R. W., Vanilovich, I., Sevkovskaya, Z., Dzikovich, I., et al. (2004). Feeding effects on growth during infancy. *Journal of Pediatrics, 145*(5), 600-605.

Kramer, M. S., & Kakuma, R. (2012). Optimal duration of exclusive breastfeeding *Cochrane Database of Systematic Reviews, Art No. CD003517.*

La Leche League International. (LLLI). (2008). *Storing human milk.* Schaumburg, IL: Author.

Lawrence, R. A., & Lawrence, R. M. (2011). *Breastfeeding: A guide for the medical profession* (7th Ed.). Philadelphia, PA: Elsevier Mosby.

Li, R., Fein, S. B., & Grummer-Strawn, L. M. (2008). Association of breastfeeding intensity and bottle-emptying behaviors at early infancy with infants' risk for excess weight at late infancy. *Pediatrics, 122 Suppl 2,* S77-84.

Li, R., Magadia, J., Fein, S. B., & Grummer-Strawn, L. M. (2012). Risk of bottle-feeding for rapid weight gain during the first year of life. *Archives of Pediatric & Adolescent Medicine, 166*(5), 431-436.

Macknin, M. L., Medendorp, S. V., & Maier, M. C. (1989). Infant sleep and bedtime cereal. *American Journal of Diseases of Children, 143*(9), 1066-1068.

Manohar, A. A., Williamson, M., & Koppikar, G. V. (1997). Effect of storage of colostrum in various containers. *Indian Pediatrics, 34*(4), 293-295.

McGovern, P., Dowd, B., Gjerdingen, D., Dagher, R., Ukestad, L., McCaffrey, D., et al. (2007). Mothers' health and work-related factors at 11 weeks postpartum. *The Annals of Family Medicine, 5*(6), 519-527.

McGovern, P., Dowd, B., Gjerdingen, D., Gross, C. R., Kenney, S., Ukestad, L., et al. (2006). Postpartum health of employed mothers 5 weeks after childbirth. *Annals of Family Medicine, 4*(2), 159-167.

McGovern, P., Dowd, B., Gjerdingen, D., Dagher, R., Ukestad, L., McCaffrey, D., et al. (2007). Mothers' health and work-related factors at 11 weeks postpartum. *Annals of Family Medicine, 5*(6), 519-527.

McKenna, J. J., & McDade, T. (2005). Why babies should never sleep alone: A review of the co-sleeping controversy in relation to SIDS, bedsharing and breast feeding. *Paediatric Respiratory Reviews, 6*(2), 134-152.

Meier, P. (1988). Bottle- and breast-feeding: Effects on transcutaneous oxygen pressure and temperature in preterm infants. *Nursing Research, 37*(1), 36-41.

Meier, P., & Anderson, G. C. (1987). Responses of small preterm infants to bottle- and breast-feeding. *MCN American Journal of Maternal Child Nursing, 12*(2), 97-105.

Meier, P., Motykowski, J. E., & Zuleger, J. L. (2004). Choosing a correctly-fitted breast shield for milk expression. *Medela Messenger, 21*, 8-9.

Mohrbacher, N. (2011). The magic number and long-term milk production. *Clinical Lactation, 2*(1), 15-18.

Mohrbacher, N. (2010). *Breastfeeding answers made simple*. Amarillo, TX: Hale Publishing.

Molbak, K., Gottschau, A., Aaby, P., Hojlyng, N., Ingholt, L., & da Silva, A. P. (1994). Prolonged breast feeding, diarrhoeal disease, and survival of children in Guinea-Bissau. *British Medical Journal, 308*(6941), 1403-1406.

Morton, J., Hall, J. Y., Wong, R. J., Thairu, L., Benitz, W. E., & Rhine, W. D. (2009). Combining hand techniques with electric pumping increases milk production in mothers of preterm infants. *Journal of Perinatology, 29*(11), 757-764.

Morton, J., Wong, R. J., Hall, J. Y., Pang, W. W., Lai, C. T., Lui, J., et al. (2012). Combining hand techniques with electric pumping increases the caloric content of milk in mothers of preterm infants. *Journal of Perinatology, 32*(10), 791-796.

Neville, M. C., Allen, J. C., Archer, P. C., Casey, C. E., Seacat, J., Keller, R. P., et al. (1991). Studies in human lactation: milk volume and nutrient composition during weaning and lactogenesis. *American Journal of Clinical Nutrition, 54*(1), 81-92.

Nichols, M. R., & Roux, G. M. (2004). Maternal perspectives on postpartum return to the workplace. *Journal of Obstetric, Gynecologic, & Neonatal Nursing, 33*(4), 463-471.

Nielsen, S. B., Reilly, J. J., Fewtrell, M. S., Eaton, S., Grinham, J., & Wells, J. C. (2011). Adequacy of milk intake during exclusive breastfeeding: A longitudinal study. *Pediatrics, 128*(4), e907-914.

NWLC. (2012). *The next generation of Title IX: Pregnant and parenting students* [Electronic Version].Retrieved from: http://www.titleix.info/history/history-overview.aspx

Odom, E. C., Li, R., Scanlon, K. S., Perrine, C. G., & Grummer-Strawn, L. (2013). Reasons for earlier than desired cessation of breastfeeding. *Pediatrics, 131*(3), e726-732.

OECD. (2011). *Health at a glance 2011: OECD Indicators: 4.9 Caesarean sections.* Retrieved from: http://www.oecd-ilibrary. org/sites/health_glance-2011-en/04/09/g4-09-01.html?itemId=/content/chapter/health_glance-2011-37-en

Ogbuanu, C., Glover, S., Probst, J., Liu, J., & Hussey, J. (2011). The effect of maternity leave length and time of return to work on breastfeeding. *Pediatrics, 127*(6), e1414-1427.

Ogbuanu, C., Glover, S., Probst, J., Hussey, J., & Liu, J. (2011). Balancing work and family: Effect of employment characteristics on breastfeeding. *Journal of Human Lactation, 27*(3), 225-238; quiz 293-225.

Ortiz, J., McGilligan, K., & Kelly, P. (2004). Duration of breast milk expression among working mothers enrolled in an employer-sponsored lactation program. *Pediatric Nursing, 30*(2), 111-119.

PAHO/WHO. (2001). *Guiding principles for complementary feeding of the breastfed child.* Retrieved from: http://whqlibdoc.who. int/paho/2004/a85622.pdf.

Paxson, C. L., Jr., & Cress, C. C. (1979). Survival of human milk leukocytes. *Journal of Pediatrics, 94*(1), 61-64.

Perrine, C. G., Scanlon, K. S., Li, R., Odom, E., & Grummer-Strawn, L. M. (2012). Baby-Friendly hospital practices and meeting exclusive breastfeeding intention. *Pediatrics, 130*(1), 54-60.

Peterson, A., & Harmer, M. (2010). *Balancing breast & bottle: Reaching your breastfeeding goals.* Amarillo, TX: Hale Publishing.

Pittard, W. B., 3rd, & Bill, K. (1981). Human milk banking. Effect of refrigeration on cellular components. *Clinical Pediatrics, 20*(1), 31-33.

Prime, D. K., Kent, J. C., Hepworth, A. R., Trengove, N. J., & Hartmann, P. E. (2012). Dynamics of milk removal during simultaneous breast expression in women. *Breastfeeding Medicine, 7*(2), 100-106.

Quan, R., Yang, C., Rubinstein, S., Lewiston, N. J., Sunshine, P., Stevenson, D. K., et al. (1992). Effects of microwave radiation on anti-infective factors in human milk. *Pediatrics, 89*(4 Pt 1), 667-669.

Rechtman, D. J., Lee, M. L., & Berg, H. (2006). Effect of environmental conditions on unpasteurized donor human milk. *Breastfeeding Medicine, 1*(1), 24-26.

Roe, B., Whittington, L. A., Fein, S. B., & Teisl, M. F. (1999). Is there competition between breast-feeding and maternal employment? *Demography, 36*(2), 157-171.

SHRM. (2013). *2012 employee benefits research report.* Retrieved from: http://www.shrm.org/research/surveyfindings/articles/pages/2012employeebenefitsresearchreport.aspx

Sievers, E., Oldigs, H. D., Santer, R., & Schaub, J. (2002). Feeding patterns in breast fed and formula-fed infants. *Annals of Nutrition and Metabolism, 46*(6), 243-248.

Skafida, V. (2012). Juggling work and motherhood: The impact of employment and maternity leave on breastfeeding duration: A survival analysis on Growing Up in Scotland data. *Maternal and Child Health Journal, 16*(2), 519-527.

Slusser, W. M., Lange, L., Dickson, V., Hawkes, C., & Cohen, R. (2004). Breast milk expression in the workplace: A look at frequency and time. *Journal of Human Lactation, 20*(2), 164-169.

Stuebe, A. M., & Rich-Edwards, J. W. (2009). The reset hypothesis: Lactation and maternal metabolism. *American Journal of Perinatology, 26*(1), 81-88.

Stuebe, A. M., Rich-Edwards, J. W., Willett, W. C., Manson, J. E., & Michels, K. B. (2005). Duration of lactation and incidence of type 2 diabetes. *Journal of the American Medical Association, 294*(20), 2601-2610.

Stuebe, A. M., & Schwarz, E. B. (2010). The risks and benefits of infant feeding practices for women and their children. *Journal of Perinatology, 30*(3), 155-162.

Takci, S., Gulmez, D., Yigit, S., Dogan, O., & Hascelik, G. (2013). Container type and bactericidal activity of human milk during refrigerated storage. *Journal of Human Lactation*, *29*(3), 406-411.

Walker, M. (2011). *Breastfeeding and employment*. Amarillo, TX: Hale Publishing.

Walsh, W. (2011). *Single babe breastfeeding: It CAN be done!* Retrieved from: http://www.bestforbabes.org/single-babe-breast feeding-it-can-be-done

Wang, W., Parker, K., & Taylor, P. (2013). *Breadwinner moms*. Washington, DC: Pew Research Center.

West, D., & Marasco, L. (2009). *The breastfeeding mother's guide to making more milk*. New York: McGraw Hill.

Williamson, M. T., & Murti, P. K. (1996). Effects of storage, time, temperature, and composition of containers on biologic components of human milk. *Journal of Human Lactation*, *12*(1), 31-35.

Wilson-Clay, B., & Hoover, K. (2008). *The breastfeeding atlas* (4th Ed.). Manchaca, TX: LactNews Press.

World Health Organization. (WHO). (2010). *Infant and young child feeding*. Retrieved from: http://www.who.int/mediacen tre/factsheets/fs342/en/index.html

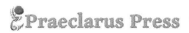
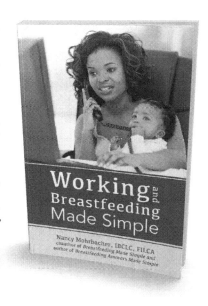

Made in the USA
Charleston, SC
13 October 2016